Early Stage Dementia

Sufferer derives from the verb 'to suffer'—French 'suffrir'; Latin 'sufferre:bear'. ie. to undergo, experience, to be subjected to, to bear with pain, loss, grief, change etc. A sufferer is one who sustains disadvantage or loss; one who endures patiently or bravely a life experience that is difficult or painful.

Early Stage Dementia
reassurance for sufferers and carers

Lorraine West

Newleaf

This book is for all those in my life who have taught me.

For more information about the author go to:
www.geocities.com/lhwestau or email her at:
lhwest@bigpond.com

Newleaf
an imprint of
Gill & Macmillan Ltd
Hume Avenue, Park West, Dublin 12
with associated companies throughout the world
www.gillmacmillan.ie
Copyright © 2001, 2003 Lorraine West
First published in Australia in 2001 by Hodder Headline Australia Pty Limited.
This Newleaf edition is published by arrangement with Hodder Headline
Australia Pty Limited.
0 7171 3567 5
Printed by ColourBooks Ltd, Dublin

The paper used in this book comes from the wood pulp of managed forests.
For every tree felled, at least one tree is planted, thereby renewing natural resources.

A CIP catalogue record for this book is available from the British Library.

1 3 5 4 2

Contents

Foreword Noreen Whittaker   vii
Preface   ix

1 Introduction   1

Part one   **Concerns about memory**

2 Pre-diagnosis   11
3 Being diagnosed   30
4 Behavioural changes   51
5 Drug treatments   59

Part two   **Living with dementia**

6 A rite of passage   72
7 Beyond the patient: partners, family and friends   81
8 The Living with Memory Loss Program   90

Part three   **The psychology of caring**

9 The family   125
10 The family system   147
11 Caring for the carer   151
12 Hidden loss   162
13 Attachment and non-attachment   172
14 Counselling   179

Part four   **Mind, body, spirit**

15 Looking after yourself   205
16 Resilience   221

Appendix I   Statistics about dementia   238
Appendix II   Diagnostic criteria for dementia of the
               Alzheimer's type   240
Appendix III   Folstein Mini Mental State Examination   242
Appendix IV   Geriatric Depression Scale   246

Notes   248
Contacts   256
Index   261
Acknowledgments   268

Beannacht [Blessing]

On the day when
the weight deadens
on your shoulders
and you stumble,
may the clay dance
to balance you.
And when your eyes
freeze behind
the grey window
and the ghost of loss
gets in to you,
may a flock of colours,
indigo, red, green
and azure blue
come to awaken in you
a meadow of delight.

When the canvas frays
in the curach of thought
and a stain of ocean
blackens beneath you,
may there come across the waters
a path of yellow moonlight
to bring you safely home.

May the nourishment of the earth be yours,
may the clarity of light be yours,
may the fluency of the ocean be yours
may the protection of the ancestors be yours.
And so may a slow
mind work these words
of love around you,
an invisible cloak
to mind your life.

'Beannacht' from *Anam Cara: Spiritual Wisdom from the Celtic World* by John O'Donohue published by Bantam Press. Used by permission of Transworld Publishers, a division of The Random House Group Limited.

Foreword

LEARNING TO UNDERSTAND AND LIVE WITH DEMENTIA CHANGES your life. There are not many life experiences that can prepare you for a journey that has no clear purpose, an uncertain destination, no defined route, or even a time frame. It is a journey that involves at least two people but usually whole families. It causes you to re-assess your own way of functioning in the world and how you handle your own emotions and those of other people.

I am a spouse of a person with dementia. My husband, Wal, has dementia of the Alzheimer's type that was diagnosed, 11 years ago when he was only 50. His symptoms presented at least two years before the cause of his dementia was diagnosed, so many of the options available to those in early stage of a dementing illness today were not available to us.

Much of this book resonates with me. As I read it, I found myself nodding knowingly, sometimes sadly, wishing that I'd had this bit of information or that perspective at the beginning of our journey and not years later after learning the hard way.

If only I knew then what I know now; how different that early stage may have been!

Learning to live with any illness can be difficult. To learn to live with one where the patient may have no visible physical disability in the early stages and can have inconsistent behaviour patterns and impaired communication skills is exceptionally hard. Not knowing what to expect nor for how long compounds the sense of panic when one is faced with the prospect of an uncertain future.

Early Stage Dementia recognises that both the carer and the affected person are equal in their need for support and understanding and that the process must commence as early as possible to be most effective.

This book not only reports on the innovative programs now available but gives valuable facts about the nature of irreversible dementia, what to expect of the condition, practical tips for management and current drug therapies. It also recounts many individual interviews with people with dementia and family members that powerfully portray personal pain and struggle as well as informative and instructive insights. Furthermore, it analyses the nature of families and their complex, overwhelming emotions. And, finally, it provides a beacon of hope in the discussion about the nature of resilience and how control can be regained.

It is a book that seeks to support and guide individuals, families and professionals as they begin a journey with dementia.

I would urge anyone who is affected by a dementing illness not to ignore the signs and symptoms and to seek help as early as possible.

And to read this book!

Noreen Whittaker

Preface

THE TIME BEFORE A PERSON IS DIAGNOSED WITH A DEMENTING illness varies from months to years; a period that can be very distressing as people try to get answers, especially if they are younger than sixty-five. Dementia is often perceived as something that only happens to very old people, so the idea of actually having a dementing illness while still at work or preparing for retirement is incomprehensible. Yet it does happen.

Although we refer to dementia as a disease it is not a physical illness; it is a syndrome or a set of symptoms caused by a whole range of degenerative illnesses. Alzheimer's disease is one such illness. Dementia affects all aspects of a person's life and eventually leads to a disconnection from self, family and friends. This process can take many, many years, but in the meantime there is much that can be done to minimise its effects. The fact that the unique needs of people with early stage dementia need recognition has only recently been acknowledged and moved into public awareness. Newly diagnosed people are no longer expected to go home and cope the best way they can. Receiving a diagnosis after many months of 'tests' frequently leaves people in a daze, followed closely by anguish, distress, feeling out of control and a loss of emotional bearings. Regaining some sense of control and direction following a diagnosis of a dementing illness can be greatly helped with the right information, emotional support, practical assistance, understanding and compassion.

This book challenges the belief that very little can be done to sustain or enhance the quality of life for the person with a dementing illness or for their carers.

Today there are programs developed specifically for people in the early stages of dementia that offer support and education. These programs allow people to share their experiences and to hear about others in a similar situation. Being offered a place to react to the diagnosis, voice their experiences and relate to others is revolutionary. In the past people were not always even informed as to what was happening to them; it was considered by some doctors to be unhelpful to offer a diagnosis as there was no medical treatment available.

One program which this book looks at is the Living with Memory Loss program. Families are invited to participate along with the person with the dementing illness; in fact, their love and support is an integral part of the overall program. It addresses the changes that occur for the person with the dementing illness and outlines adaptations that the family have to make. This program is innovative, inclusive and educational and provides a place where the changes that are occurring in the family can be spoken about in a non-judgmental environment. The essence of the program is for the person with the dementing illness to be understood, and for the family to understand the changes in a supportive environment.

People with dementia of the Alzheimer's type can now be offered drug treatments that slow down the process of the illness. While this is not a cure, it is most definitely a step in the right direction and more drugs are now being trialled. It is advisable that people who are worried about changes in their memory, their work habits, their moods or their behaviour seek advice and assessment from their doctor, as these drugs are recommended for people in the early to moderate stages of dementia rather than the later stages.

The family is now included in both care and treatments from the point of diagnosis. Counselling with a therapist trained in all aspects of dementia care is offered to people in the early stages of dementia and beyond. Counselling provides another avenue of support that addresses the collective and individual needs of each person in the family. In the following pages I will expand upon the role of the family and the carer, and how the carer can remain connected to both the person with the illness and to themselves.

Good care is a combination of four concurrent pathways: the comprehensive medical assessment and diagnosis; the commencement of drug treatment (if appropriate); participation in a Living with Memory Loss group or another early intervention support group; and individual or family counselling. These options do not always follow in sequential order, but it is essential that early diagnosis be the first step; the others will follow. There is no need for people to keep quiet and suffer alone any more.

This book will explain how each of these four main pathways interface with each other and help demystify the journey for those people newly diagnosed and for families and friends who choose to be involved in this journey.

My wish is that people will no longer be so frightened they deny that there is a problem and fail to seek appropriate help when they are concerned about cognitive and behavioural changes. In the not too distant future people will be offered treatment a long time before any observable changes have occurred in their brain scans. So what is known today as early stage dementia will move to a different position on the continuum of care. Scientists and researchers are working to find a cure but in the meantime much can be done, and there are many avenues of support and help available.

I write with confidence and optimism about what is currently available to enable people to make informed choices about their lives, and hope that this book will help to demystify the process. Some of the material in this book has been obtained from interviews both with people with a dementing illness and their families. These very kind people have agreed to share part of their story in the hope that others will have a less arduous journey. Names and identifying information have been changed to protect their privacy.

1 Introduction

DEMENTIA HAS BEEN EVIDENT IN SOCIETY FOR CENTURIES. IT HAS often been depicted in both art and film in its most negative manifestation. All too frequently, the artist's impression, the film director's imagination and the actor's interpretation of dementia are at best overemphasised or grossly exaggerated. In the box office hit film *Amadeus*, for instance, Antonio Salieri, while sitting behind a baby grand piano in a mental asylum in Vienna, tells the tale of his musical demise caused by Wolfgang Mozart. He is surrounded by tortured souls, half naked, tied to walls with chains, while he muses over his losses and weeps for his own self-described mediocrity. Later, Mozart is immortalised for his genius, and Salieri is left alone to ungraciously perish.

The scriptwriters never attempted to segregate fiction from truth; the negative depictions of dementia and madness remain in people's minds. And after more than two hundred years of such distortions, fear of mental illness is widespread in our society. Families of many people recently diagnosed with dementia are fearful of the stigma that surrounds anything to do with the mind and of how society will treat them differently. Some people still believe that dementia is catching.

Carers interviewed for this book offered insights into why disclosing the diagnosis of dementia would cause them additional distress:

> *We didn't tell many relatives about my husband's diagnosis of dementia. Again, that decision was based on the fact they would treat him differently…I wanted to cover it up. It's not like having heart disease, this is the mind. I did not want to be treated differently either.*
>
> *I was concerned about protecting him. I was concerned as to how the diagnosis of this illness would be perceived. It could have been seen as an infectious or contagious mental illness…those sorts of perceptions.*

Today dementia is managed very differently to how it was in the past—while not curable, it is certainly treatable. The majority of changes have slowly evolved over the past ten years. Only recently has attention been given to the early stage of dementia, a crucial time for positive changes to be integrated. The maintenance of a purposeful life, friendships, family relationships and connections to those who are important to us is essential while living with memory problems.

There are currently nearly 18 million people with dementia worldwide. Dementia affects all aspects of a person's life and eventually leads to a disconnection with the self, family and friends. Until recently it was incorrectly believed that as there was no medical cure for dementia nothing could be done, and people were prematurely abandoned both physically and psychologically. We are talking about an illness with around ten to fifteen years' duration, an incredible amount of time to be set apart from family and society.

Although there are many causes of a dementing illness, the majority of people diagnosed will be suffering from Alzheimer's disease or have some form of vascular dementia. Dementia is not a disease in its own right. The dementing illness will be characterised by an impairment of memory, abstract thinking and judgment, changes in personality and a reduction in previous occupational and/or social functioning.

The word dementia is derived from the Latin *de*, meaning 'from' and *mentis*, meaning 'mind'. Alzheimer's disease is named after a German neurologist, Alois Alzheimer, who described its characteristics in 1907. It is a progressive disease accompanied by microscopic structural changes in the brain. These changes can occur in older persons without dementia, but it is the intensity of the degeneration that distinguishes Alzheimer's disease from normal ageing.[1] The actual cause of Alzheimer's disease is as yet unknown.

Dementia is most usually a disease of old age, but old age does not necessarily result in dementia. However, you don't have to be old to have dementia; it is estimated that there are 18,500 people under the age of sixty-five with dementia in the UK. Those aged above sixty have a one in ten chance of developing Alzheimer's disease and a one in four chance over eighty years of age. Between 1995 and 2041 the number of people with dementia is expected to rise by 254 per cent because people are living longer.[2] Studies in the USA estimate that dementing illnesses now affect more than four million people.

Changes to a person's memory, mood, behaviour and the level of competence with which they conduct their activities of daily living or their occupation are the first signs that something has changed or is changing.

We have all forgotten something important at various times. We do not like forgetting things, as it can convey to others a sense of us being incompetent, or lacking concentration, even being irresponsible. The result may be self-criticism, embarrassment, inconvenience, or a feeling of being out of control.

What is memory?

Short-term memory is the ability to recall a recent visit of a friend or a message being given or someone phoning to say hello. Finding a telephone number to make a phone call is a normal everyday event, but unless we repeat or learn the phone number off by heart it will be forgotten very quickly. Problems with short-term memory cause untold distress, because short-term memory is what we use to negotiate our way through life and maintain our independence.

Long-term memory is recalling events or telling stories about childhood experiences in the distant past. Information that has been well processed and integrated into one's general knowledge store remains intact for some people with a dementing illness for a long time,[3] so they can continue to feel useful and valued for many years.

The following pages do not prescribe treatment; instead, they offer an alternative approach to the early stages of dementia. This will hopefully influence a shift in thinking about a subject that will affect us all, in some way, as our population ages.

The introduction provides a historical overview of the technological, statistical projections of dementia sufferers, as well as the psychosocial changes that have occurred around the world over the past twenty years, including changes to the care of people with dementia.

Part one describes dementia in general, including the changes that are first noticed, the value of a diagnosis and frequently asked questions; an outline of the process of obtaining a diagnosis; discussion of the issues relating to disclosing the diagnosis; resources available at the time of diagnosis; changes to the brain that cause the behavioural changes; and progress in new treatments for dementia.

Part two discusses living with dementia; how the changes affect partners, family and friends; outcomes from equal involvement; and the role of memory loss programs.

Part three gives insight into the psychology of self and others; why we feel and react the way we do; and how solutions to problems within families can be addressed.

Part four offers a process by which family carers can move from a position of adversity to one of resilience and mastery over their own lives. It demonstrates how redefinition of the self and a reinvestment in life can be achieved.

Explanation of terms

Early stage dementia

Early stage dementia is a term used to describe the period preceding, and for some period after, diagnosis. If the dementing illness is not complicated by other diseases, a person in the early stages will require very little assistance with self-care activities, such as showering, dressing and personal grooming. Most people in the early stages are very aware of the problems they are having with their memory and cognitive functions; it is only in the latter stages of dementia that people can lose awareness of their cognitive and physical losses. The age of the person with early stage dementia is significant. If a person is employed with a family still at home a very different set of adjustments will be necessary from those of a person who is retired.

The term 'early stage' is at best only a guide as there is no definitive line between the early or beginning stages of the disease. Influencing factors may be the person's social situation, the exact nature of the dementing illness, the age of onset, the areas in which a person can still function successfully, and other illnesses. The degree of support from the family is important, as it is the family that has the ability to reduce anxiety and to assist the person to maximise their cognitive capacities.

Carer

The word *carer* does not necessarily mean a relative; rather, it is the person that has chosen to be in partnership with the person with

dementia and views care from the position of protection, consideration, serious attention and commitment. Furthermore, a carer can be
any person who has a positive attachment to the person with dementia:
a grandchild, friend, spouse, son, daughter, mother, father, sister, brother
or neighbour. The word carer is used in this book despite the fact that
there has been much debate occurring around the notion of what
being a carer is. For some it can be the primary reason for one's existence, while others see it as a normal part of a relationship. Still others
reject the role but undertake it as a sense of duty. Generally, there will
be a primary caregiver of the person with dementia whatever their
relationship or motivation. It is my belief that the role of carer should
be viewed in equal partnership with the person with dementia for the
duration of the disease. This perspective needs to be maintained by
all those who will be involved.

Other terms

The term *person with a dementing illness* is used interchangeably with
person with dementia. The word *patient* is used where a medical research
paper has used the same term. *Family member* is used but does not
necessarily mean that the family member is involved in the care. Instead,
they might have a position of influence in terms of the impact of
dementia upon the family. The *client* is the person who seeks assistance from the Alzheimer's Association. The term *group participants*
automatically includes both people diagnosed with dementia and carers.
They attend the group program as a 'couple' then separate into their
respective groups, as their needs are very different.

The journey of dementia starts from the position of sufferers being
reasonably stable and in control of their lives, and works towards
preparing them for being totally destabilised and disconnected with
the world. The goal is to provide comfort, understanding, insight and
hope.

I have maintained the practical or clinical side of dementia because it's real, it's what I know, and I have an in-depth understanding growing from my training and history. Long ago a tutor of mine planted the seeds of this different perspective for dealing with people who had a mental illness. After some years working in this field, these seeds have germinated and provided me with additional knowledge, which I would like to share with you. Providing practical guidance to people with a dementing illness and their carers will enable them to develop alternative ways of coping with the complex and idiosyncratic disease they will encounter. The aim is for people to gain a sense of mastery about what is happening, and a sense of hope about their ability to cope with the future.

part one

Concerns about memory

2 Pre-diagnosis

THE TIME BEFORE A PERSON IS DIAGNOSED WITH DEMENTIA VARIES from months to years. This period can be very distressing as people try to get answers to problems through a variety of media, especially if they are younger than sixty-five. For most people, the idea of actually having a dementing illness while still working or in the process of winding down from their work is incomprehensible. In an attempt to make sense of changes that are occurring either to themselves or to a family member, people have sought answers from doctors, acupuncturists, herbalists, massage therapists, physiotherapists and counsellors.

Dementia is often perceived as something that happens to very old people who no longer require the same things or have the same responsibilities as in the past. Whatever avenue is taken by families in attempting to fix the problem will require understanding and compassion.

Early warning signs

The term 'early stage dementia' is generally used to describe those first symptoms early in the illness that are of concern but which generally enable normal or near normal function either at home or at work.

Memory problems alert people to the fact that something is not quite right. Anxiety, confusion or fear often inhibit a person from telling others that they are worried about themselves or are seeking a diagnosis. The person may become irritable or angry for no apparent reason. One carer recalled, 'He was angry but it was a frustrated anger—he would fly off the handle at things that normally wouldn't have worried him.' In such instances people would be more likely to search for historical triggers such as work or a problem within the family rather than consider a cognitive disorder or organic disease as the cause.

Alzheimer's disease is the major cause of dementia but it is not the only disease to cause dementia—there are actually over 100 illnesses contributing to what we know as dementia. Each person is different, but the symptoms listed in Table 2.1 are usually present.

Table 2.1
Ten early warning signs of Alzheimer's disease[1]

- Recent memory loss
- Difficulty performing familiar tasks
- Language problems
- Time and place disorientation
- Loss of judgment
- Problems with abstract thinking
- Misplacing things
- Changes in mood or behaviour
- Changes in personality
- Loss of initiative

Of course, anyone can experience any of these symptoms in their life, but there is a difference between normal forgetfulness and the signs of dementia.[2]

Recent memory loss

This may affect job skills; forgetting an assignment, a business phone number or appointment, but remembering it later, are all normal forgetfulness. The person with dementia may forget these things more often and rarely remember them later.

People who suffer problems with their memory can come from all walks of life: tradespeople, doctors, teachers, pilots, administrators, council workers, writers, dancers, technicians, scientists, journalists, nurses, television producers, engineers, social workers and housewives. They can come from a wide range of different family structures: traditional or nuclear, stepfamilies or blended families, single parent families, gay or lesbian families and extended families where two or three generations all live under the one roof. Memory problems do not discriminate against race, culture, class, gender, political affiliations or age groups. They can occur in people who may be working or semi-retired and in those with disabilities, other illnesses or in robust health.

Difficulty performing familiar tasks

Normal forgetfulness might have you doing too many things at once so you leave the carrots on the stove and serve them at the end of the meal. With dementia, you prepare the meal but forget to serve it, and might even forget having made it. You go to mow the lawn, only to return saying that the lawnmower doesn't work. You might go back to try two or three times before someone intervenes and finds that the equipment works just fine.

Language problems

Sometimes you might have trouble finding the right word and use two or three words to explain yourself. The person with dementia forgets simple words or says completely wrong words and so might sound unfathomable.

Time and place disorientation

You sometimes forget the day of the week, especially if you're on holiday or retired, or you might forget what you have to do and when, for a moment. The person with dementia can get lost in their own street not knowing where they are, how they arrived there or how to get back. They can get lost right outside their own house.

Loss of judgment

In normal circumstances you might temporarily forget the child you are watching, especially if the phone rings or you are otherwise distracted. A person with dementia can forget entirely the child in their care and go down the street to the shops, unaware that they are leaving the child behind. They can completely forget to collect a child from school, even if they've been performing this task for the last year or so.

Problems with abstract thinking

Anyone can find balancing a bank account difficult when it is more complicated than usual, especially when the system alters as with, for example, changes in taxation or welfare systems. A person with dementia has difficulty learning anything that is new, for example, how to operate a computer, obtaining their money from automatic teller machines, or following a street directory in an unfamiliar suburb.

Misplacing things

At sometime or another everyone temporarily misplaces items such as handbags, sunglasses, shopping lists or the hammer. A person with dementia puts things in inappropriate places, such as leaving their hammer in the bathroom cabinet or their shaver in the cutlery drawer.

Changes in mood or behaviour

Normally, your personality changes slowly over time. Everyone experiences mood changes, for example, if you're excited or anticipating something positive your mood tends to lighten, or if you see a sad movie you can become pensive or reflective. You respond appropriately to the event. A person with dementia won't take in all of the contextual meaning of the film, may be left unaffected by its emotional content and might laugh in the wrong places. Conversely, uncontrolled crying and depression are common moods in people with dementia.

Changes in personality

Flexibility is often one of the hallmarks of maturity. As you age you are more able to compromise and become more accepting and non-judgmental. A person with dementia may have a complete personality change, becoming suspicious or apprehensive, or flat, apathetic and uncommunicative. They might go from being a person who is gentle and unassuming to a person who is intermittently aggressive. On the other hand, they may change from someone who is fiery to someone who is compliant and malleable.

Loss of initiative

At times normal people may tire of housework, business or social life—you do not fire on twelve cylinders every single day. You fluctuate in your energy levels depending on other circumstances occurring in your life such as health, finances, responsibilities and stress. The person with dementia becomes unable to take initiative for housework tasks or business decisions. They become very passive and need to be encouraged to become involved in daily activities. They cease to initiate social and personal contacts, not phoning friends, perhaps not kissing their spouse goodbye as they leave the house.

As stated previously, dementia is a broad term used to describe a loss or impairment of a person's ability to use their brain. The most common feature is the loss of intellectual abilities, which interferes with a person's socialisation, daily living or occupation. Some people show evidence of delirium, which is clouding of one's consciousness, leading at times to confusion and/or difficulty in sustaining attention or focus. Memory impairment may be present but this could be caused by the delirium and not by the dementia.

Irreversible dementias include Alzheimer's disease, Pick's disease, multi-infarct dementia, Creutzfeldt-Jakob disease, Kuru, general paresis, Parkinson's disease, Huntingtons disease, Wilson's disease and Binswanger's disease.

Reversible conditions

Some conditions that cause dementia can be treated and therefore reverse the dementia; these are listed in Table 2.2.

The pre-diagnosis period

The events and changes in the life of a person with early stage dementia who has yet to be diagnosed are generally only recognised as significant in retrospect. Something might happen that is slotted into the basket called 'Yes, but we all do that sometimes' and is promptly forgotten. It is only when a second or third incident occurs, or maybe someone at work or home makes a comment about a behaviour, mood or loss of a skill, that medical help is sought. Then the often lengthy process of testing, waiting, testing and waiting commences.

Often the changes that are being experienced occur infrequently. An appointment, a word, a family member's name or the car registration number may be forgotten. These things can be brushed aside and rationalised when a diagnosis has not yet been reached. The time it takes to confirm the diagnosis of Alzheimer's disease can be very tough and trying and is often not duly considered by carers and health professionals. The inability to receive answers to the questions many people have about their condition and to understand what is happening to them can lead to feelings of isolation and helplessness. The experience of feeling that they are not in control of themselves, especially in social situations or at work, added to the fear of a diagnosis,

Table 2.2

Reversible causes of dementia and delirium[3]

	Delirium	Dementia
Depression		Yes
Congestive heart failure	Yes	Yes
Acute myocardial infarct	Yes	
Renal failure	Yes	Yes
Hypoglycaemia	Yes	Yes
Hyperglycaemia	Yes	Yes
Hypothyroidism	Yes	Yes
Hyperthyroidism	Yes	Yes
Pneumonia	Yes	
Diverticulitis	Yes	
Transient ischaemia	Yes	
Stroke	Yes	Yes
Subdural haematoma	Yes	Yes
Concussion	Yes	
Neurosyphilis	Yes	Yes
Tuberculosis	Yes	Yes
Brain tumour	Yes	Yes
Brain abscess	Yes	Yes
Normal pressure hydrocephalus (abnormal flow of spinal fluid)		Yes
Faecal impaction	Yes	
Urinary retention	Yes	
Sensory deprivation states (such as blindness or deafness)	Yes	Yes
Environmental changes and isolation	Yes	Yes
Electrolyte abnormalities		Yes
Lifelong alcoholism		Yes
Anaemia	Yes	Yes
Chronic lung disease with hypoxia	Yes	Yes
Deficiencies of nutrients (such as vitamins B12, folic acid, niacin)		Yes
Drug intoxication	Yes	Yes*
Bladder or urinary tract infection	Yes	

amounts to a traumatic time for both the sufferer and their families. Consider the comments of one child about her father's changed behaviour:

He went on about stupid things that no one really cared about; 'he went on about toilet rolls.' He said, 'Don't use the whole roll; just use two leaves.' We weren't told when it actually started. It kind of made it a bit hard because we did not know if he was doing something normal or something strange. But you could definitely tell he was doing something different to the way he was meant to do it. We knew his doctor was treating him for depression.

When we were really young he would take us to the park. He used to pick us up and swing us on the willow trees, and that was really nice but it doesn't make any sense now. He now feels a need to control other people because he can't control himself. The other day we had a friend over for lunch and he said, 'Sit over the plate, don't spill things down your front,' and just yelled and yelled at her. I said quietly to my friend, 'Don't worry about it. He can't face change.' Like if we are going to change house he can't cope, we can't renovate. When we bought the computer he said, 'Look at all those cables—you will blow up the house.'

He hurts you emotionally. When someone else's dad yells it's just a normal routine, but when Dad yells it is like you are being bashed. He yells at Mum and tells her that it is all her fault. He hurts you by what he says and how he says it. Verbal bullying.

This child is experiencing major behavioural changes in her father and trying valiantly to adapt and to cope with this uninvited event in her young life. The impact of these changes on her father's personality is experienced both in the privacy of her home and at school. The child becomes the advocate for her father's behaviour when her friends are embarrassed, soothing them with reassurances such as, 'Dad did not mean to do that, he is okay. Come outside and we can play there.' This has a substantial effect on the emotional development of the child, who is forced to become a carer herself at a young age.

The experience with Alzheimer's disease is a stop-start, slow, erratic dance that does not make any sense at the time. The person who has the symptoms will also often resort to coping behaviours that they have used successfully in the past. Some will try and manage the problem privately, others will seek out advice and then think about taking action, while others will tell a partner or friend and request confidentiality. These responses are all quite normal. As the friend of one person with early stage dementia said:

> *After our golf game on Saturday, Ben told me of an incident at work where he had forgotten to include all the employees' fringe benefits in a spreadsheet. He was with a bunch of company auditors and he felt such an idiot that he wished the floor could have opened up and swallowed him.*

Human nature intervenes when we are confronted with a fear or by a new situation. We take the experience on board and try to make sense or meaning of it in our own time. The situation is often linked to a past experience. This natural process of slowly turning to face a situation rather than accepting it immediately is unfairly called 'denial', or putting your head in the sand. However, it serves the purpose of letting a person adjust to the changes gradually and helps them to eventually cope in a positive way.

In the period of time between when a person first starts suffering symptoms and when they seek a diagnosis, situations occur that can often be detrimental to the sufferer. It is only with hindsight that a person can make sense of their actions and accept those situations and reclaim their dignity. This reflection on past events before diagnosis is often painful but necessary for sufferers when considering how they might handle similar situations in the future.

Many people with Alzheimer's disease later clearly remember the changes in mood and concentration, getting lost and forgetting familiar things. This pre-diagnosis or pre-clinical stage is often remembered as an extremely traumatic time in their lives. Experts in the field are now strongly suggesting that if people are worried about their memory they should do something immediately. If the memory lapses are not caused by dementia but are connected with other health or life-stage issues, the difficulties can be addressed and in some cases reversed.

Younger onset dementia

There are two very different categories for the pre-diagnosis period: younger onset dementia in those younger than sixty-five years of age, and dementia in people over sixty-five years of age. In the younger onset category, people are being diagnosed in their thirties, forties and fifties. Many are still in the workforce with a mortgage and often have young children at home. Their needs and the burden of their illness on their families and carers are likely to be very different from those people who develop dementia much later in life.

The pre-diagnosis period is a time when a person experiences changes that appear uncharacteristic or different. Pre-diagnosis can take anywhere from a few months to ten years. Some sufferers retrospectively confirm that they noticed changes up to ten years prior to the diagnosis but had put it down to other causes, especially when the person is young. As one carer of her 47-year-old husband said:

> *He was being treated for depression by our GP and he was off work for a couple of weeks. He was then referred to a psychiatrist, who treated him for depression for a long period of time. The psychiatrist then sent him to a neuropsychologist for testing. He was given a provisional diagnosis of frontal lobe dementia. He*

needed to have a CT scan and that would take another eight months.

Thinking back, little things started changing about five or six years before the diagnosis. Like, he stopped playing cricket and cards—which he was very good at. He just decided to stop.

It is most likely that people will initially look for excuses such as a mid-life crisis, early menopause, stress or depression for uncharacteristic changes. They will, not unreasonably, apportion blame to changes that may be occurring in the workplace or to some life event within the family involving a loss such as a death, a child leaving home, a divorce, unplanned retrenchment or retirement. The following comments came from the carers of dementia sufferers in their late forties or early fifties.

We had a neighbour who was doing alterations to his house next door. Council approved, no big deal. I mean, you live in a society where everything is changing all of the time and if someone wants to alter a roofline a bit and put on another room, well then okay. All [my wife] could focus on was the house next door. Every day she would show me the changes to the building. It became so bad, so bad that in the end we sold the house. At the time I thought that it was all because of that damn neighbour.

I guess to be succinct, and there were many things, but it was [my husband's] lack of curiosity and spontaneity. And then there was a basic lack of drive in him which I tried to put down to tiredness or the stress of a very busy job, combined with building a house.

[Dad] wasn't as friendly. He never seemed to be excited about anything...I thought that maybe he had reached the time in his life when he was just not the same. I just thought that he was having a crisis and a bit of burn out.

[My wife] was periodically getting the bus in the wrong direction. It was not bothering her. She just said she was 'making friends with the bus driver'. I did not see these incidents as part of a pattern at that stage.

Migraines. Feeling stressed out. And I could not remember which turn to take on the way to work. I just felt that there was too much going on really. If I had not had the migraine then I would have been fired from work. I had made a few mistakes.

It started off with an anxiety problem, nervousness and also an obsession about things. Something that you or I would push away as unimportant with no consequence. To [my wife] it became an issue.

[Mum] used to forget appointments with people, but nothing major, and nothing that you would think anything of, just a bad day.

And while I was away on holiday…things went wrong with [my husband's] eyes, and mind and body and everything fell apart physically…and I kept taking him to the doctor and things were looked at but nothing was ever diagnosed or decided upon.

Early stage dementia over the age of sixty-five

The danger for sufferers over sixty-five is that changes in behaviour are more likely to be regarded as the result of pre-existing physical health issues such as conditions causing pain, poor vision or poor hearing, or of emotional issues such as the loss of a loved animal or some other form of loss, even living alone after the death of a partner. Symptoms are often seen as just being part of getting older and becoming less interested in social and family affairs.

Each pre-diagnosis period is unique and unpredictable and can be influenced either positively or negatively by people's beliefs about dementia. For people in the older age bracket, the belief that most often hinders diagnosis is that dementia is simply a part of ageing for which there is no cure. Sufferers and families, then, are less likely to seek help in the early stages. The following comments are taken from interviews with people with dementia and their partners over the age of sixty-five.

Apart from my father's basic forgetfulness, we both put that down to his age.

But I did think it was obvious that she had a failing memory, but I did not take it seriously. She was completely rational and that sort of thing except for her failing memory. We used to have a professor at college who forgot where he lived—well, I thought that was unusual, but that is all.

I just thought, oh well, you can't remember everything in life.

Just kept repeating things; it is not unusual in elderly people.

He could not remember the names of his grandchildren or sometimes his own children. It became a game when he started giving them numbers. We all just played the game—it was quite sweet. He had done that for years actually.

She was slowly going deaf and she used to ask us to repeat things, or to speak up and we all just did it . . . until she started to phone us like ten to fourteen times a day!!! Then we thought it might be something other than her hearing.

Irrespective of the event that finally attracts the attention of the person with dementia or causes someone else to seek medical help, it is important that people do not judge themselves too harshly. There are many reasons why people do not see or want to see problematical situations. The time will come when a change in behaviour, mood or functionality can no longer be ignored. What is imperative is that a full assessment be sought, irrespective of age. Being told that 'it is just part of ageing and you have to learn to live with it' is not acceptable.

Depression or dementia?

Everyone's moods change from time to time as a reaction to events in everyday life; feelings of sadness, rejection or loneliness are part of the normal spectrum of emotions. When these feeling persist or increase and are linked with other signs and symptoms that affect a person's thinking, ability to work or interest in life, it is not unusual to suspect that the cause might lie in a depressive illness. To further confuse the issue, depression can manifest as dementia while, conversely, dementia can often present with depressive symptoms in the early stages. In addition, it has been found that 30 per cent of newly diagnosed people are clinically depressed, and a further 63 per cent self diagnose as depressed.[4]

We live in a world that praises and acknowledges perfection. Physical problems such as arthritis, cardiac surgery, hip replacements, gastric ulcers and so forth can be openly discussed with family and friends as they are generally ascribed to situations above and beyond your control. But to feel anxious and flat when there is no observable cause receives much less sympathy, so people are more likely to keep quiet about feeling depressed for a long period of time. In fact, living with depression can become a way of life. Behavioural changes in a person can initially be rationalised, for example, 'She hasn't been the same since her daughter died last year,' and therefore go unnoticed and undiagnosed.

Depression may be noticed by another person, or may be identified by an astute doctor who is seeing a patient for another matter.

Minor or *reactive depression* is a normal emotional response to a loss that can be resolved often without treatment if the person is supported appropriately, allowed time to grieve, or seeks the support of a counsellor. A *major* or *clinical depression,* which can appear out of the blue, is caused by a chemical imbalance in the brain and usually responds well to anti-depressant medication and psychotherapy.

The signs and symptoms of depression include:

- feeling sad, or empty;
- diminished pleasure or interest in most day-to-day activities;
- a change in appetite—a significant weight loss or weight gain;
- changes in sleep patterns;
- fatigue—a loss of energy and sparkle;
- feelings of worthlessness;
- a reduced ability to think or concentrate;
- indecisiveness;
- a lack of expression and reactions;
- disruption to social and occupational functioning;
- crying;
- slow movements; and
- monotonous speech.

Depression may be triggered by a crisis; a loss of a person, place, object or animal; excessive stress; physical or chemical changes in your body; changes in your lifestyle; physical illness; or chronic pain. Depression tends to be an early, rather than a late feature of dementia. Perhaps it is the body's response to the growing awareness that there are problems with memory, the learning of new tasks, and the ability to manage your life as well as you did previously.

Therefore, those diagnosed with depression in later life, even if their initial symptoms respond well to treatment, need to be rigorously supervised.

Frequently asked questions

Why are symptoms not noticed much earlier?

People often do not recognise the first symptoms of dementia. They will only seek help when they cannot manage at home or work or they are having relationship difficulties. They will change jobs, take a holiday or do something to try and problem solve in the best way they know how. Often the onset is a slow process and the person with dementia fluctuates between normal or characteristic behaviour and abnormal behaviour, which can be either overt or covert. An older person in the early stages can disguise symptoms by relying on other people for answers to questions, for example, by saying to a partner, 'You know' or 'You remember'. The family can then unconsciously fall into a support position. Often memory problems are not noticed until a person is alone and gets lost or fails to do something that would be taken as normal, such as going to a place that they have been many times before.

What should a person do if they are worried about their own memory or that of another person in the family?

Seek help as early as possible. Tell your doctor what is happening and what you have felt or noticed that has changed. Generally, the doctor will refer you to a memory clinic, a neurologist, a psychogeriatrician or a geriatrician, depending on the situation. The advantage of a memory clinic is that all the necessary tests are done at the hospital and a team that specialises in dementia analyses the test results. Dementia is not a new disease, but the diagnosis is important in terms of management and ongoing review and treatment regimes.

How should the person showing symptoms be approached?

Gently and sensitively. Most people know that something is wrong and are often frightened, or may have been coping through the use of diaries and lists of things to do for some time and have not chosen to tell anyone. This fear can be seen or heard almost daily; when people forget something they will often jokingly make some reference to Alzheimer's disease or old-timer's disease.

How do you support the person with the memory problems if they are reluctant to seek help?

If at all possible admit to your own fear about them. Rather than say, 'I think that you have a problem with your memory that requires help', you could begin by expressing some of your concerns about their memory and say how you will be prepared to assist them in having some tests done. Offer your love and support and tell them that you will be there for them. Reassurance that they are not alone goes a long way to engendering confidence; it can also be a time to reflect on your own feelings about dementia. What does this mean for you? And how do you see yourself in the future if this person has dementia?

When do you tell people about your concerns?

This depends on your relationship to the person. If it is a partner, ask them what they want. Do they want others to know about your concerns, or to keep it private for the time being? If it is a parent, the same applies. The person with dementia has a choice about when or if to tell someone. If it is you, yourself, you could speak with a friend whom you trust and then seek out professional information from the help line of the Alzheimer's Association in your city.

What if the family do not want to know about the memory problem?

A good question is, 'What purpose does this denial serve?' Is there an existing illness in the family? Has there been another person in the family with dementia? Is there a cultural belief about dementia such as madness and shame?

Often the underpinning for people not wanting to know about the memory problem will be some form of fear, the exact nature of which may never be known. People will do what they can and coercion or manipulation is not advisable. It is better to have volunteers by choice than people conscripted, both for the person with the dementia and for those that are carers.

If people are worried about their memory should they tell anyone or just wait and see?

One of the reasons for informing selected people would be that others could understand the changes that are occurring in the person. In some circumstances there is a duty of care, especially for workplace situations. For example, for a nurse, doctor, forklift driver, engineer or lawyer, short-term memory loss would affect the cognitive functioning in their place of work.

How would I know if I was getting dementia because sometimes I forget things?

Forgetting things at times is pretty normal. It is persistent forgetting, reduction or loss in the ability to perform routine tasks, impairment of judgment, mood changes and/or changes in personality, difficulty in learning new tasks and the loss of some language skills that signal the possibility of Alzheimer's disease. If you are worried about any of the above symptoms it would be useful to keep a daily journal of your concerns. If the symptoms persist, go and see your doctor and talk about your concerns.

There is dementia in my family—how likely am I to get it?

Family history of Alzheimer's disease does not necessarily mean that you will get it, but it is thought to increase the chances. If a person has a first-degree blood relative with the disease they are about one and a half to two times as likely to develop Alzheimer's as those without a family history of it. Some studies have identified a genetic link in families who get the disease before the age of sixty-five; this is a rare form, or inherited 'younger onset' form.

How do you get a referral to the appropriate medical specialist?

Your local doctor is your first port of call. They will do some basic testing and may or may not refer the patient to a doctor that specialises in dementia. There are many issues that need to be considered when people are concerned about their memory, or that of another person.

They may have other illnesses that co-exist with the memory problems that require specialist intervention. Your local doctor should weigh up all the pros and cons of the situation and refer appropriately. Shared case management is now common practice among general practitioners and specialists.

Writing down a list of questions before you see your doctor is helpful, especially if you are concerned about your memory. Jotting down points as you think of them is better than trying to rely on your memory when you are sitting in the surgery.

3 Being diagnosed

THE VALUE OF GETTING A DIAGNOSIS IS HIGHLY RECOMMENDED FOR the following reasons:

- To rule out the possibility of any other physical and mental illness, including depression, which could then be treated appropriately.
- To get help, including appropriate medical treatment, as soon as possible.
- To have as many options and choices at your disposal for the management of dementia.
- To be able to plan and make informed decisions about your life, work, legal and financial affairs and housing.
- To know what kind of dementia it is and, if possible, what part of the brain is affected.
- To identify your cognitive strengths and weaknesses.
- To help your own understanding of your changed behaviour.
- To assist those who care for you to understand these changes.
- To enable you to have a choice about participation in valuable research studies.[1]

The medical community is still learning so much about dementia. Receiving a diagnosis of Alzheimer's disease means you can have a choice about participation in research studies and whether to help others in similar situations.

Assessment

There is no single test that will accurately diagnose dementia. Diagnosis is a process that may take months of gathering copious amounts of information, doing tests, often repeating tests and being referred to various specialists. A crucial part of the whole process is an attempt to exclude the likelihood of other diseases. Doctors are cautious about disclosing a diagnosis of an illness that will have a dementing component until other diseases have been ruled out. The tests do not require hospitalisation as a rule, unless a person is in hospital for another reason and is exhibiting symptoms of a dementing illness.

Assessment for a diagnosis may have several components:

- A thorough medical checkup by a general practitioner (GP).
- A neurological examination by a specialist physician, neurologist, geriatrician or psychogeriatrician.
- Psychometric testing by a neuropsychologist.
- People may be referred to a memory disorders unit in their capital city where all the tests are done at the same place.

The GP plays a pivotal role not only in the diagnosis, but in providing ongoing care and support for the person with dementia and their family. Not all doctors are specialists in dementia; while they will do the basic tests, they may then refer the patient on to a specialist.

People concerned about their memory and wishing to obtain a diagnosis can ask for a referral to a specialist at the outset. They may later work with their own doctor, who will have the specialist report on file. Most doctors will readily refer you for a specialised consultation.

The presence of memory loss, or a decrease in a previous level of functioning, should always be taken seriously by an individual's GP. Often the person having the problem is not aware of the extent or the effect that it is having on themselves or the family. It is essential, if this is the case, to take a family member along to any doctor's appointment or to have a letter written to the doctor before the visit outlining the issues if a support person is unavailable. Some doctors will request to see the family member and the patient separately.

The initial consultations

The doctor will ask the person with the symptoms (if appropriate) or a family member to describe what has been happening and what changes they have noticed. If the patient is unable to answer any questions fully then a family member or a good friend may assist by filling in missing pieces of information. Some of the typical questions that could be asked include:

- What were the first problems that you noticed, or were observed by a family member?
- Did it start gradually or suddenly?
- When was this first noticed?
- Does the problem happen occasionally, or is the frequency increasing?
- Have you ever had memory problems that you thought were more than the normal forgetfulness that we all have from time to time?
- Have you noticed problems with your work or around the home— problems relating to your thinking, or getting things in order?
- Have you had problems with your language?

- Have you had a change in your mood?
- Have you ever felt depressed?
- Have you ever had unusual thoughts—about people, places and things?
- Have you lost interest in things around you?
- Have you had any changes to your sexual interest?
- What are you most worried about?
- Has there been any major event in the family or at work in the past two years that you think could be contributing to your memory problems?[2]

The doctor may also ask questions about how the patient manages their finances, or if the family has been contacted frequently when the patient has lost house keys or experienced other difficulties.

Cognitive testing

At this point the GP may conduct an informal screening test known as the Folstein Mini Mental State Examination (MMSE, see Appendix III), which can indicate the presence of cognitive impairment. This is a short test that asks a variety of questions regarding the year, date, season, day, month and where the individual is now. It also involves writing a simple sentence, copying a drawing and a short task completion exercise. Attention, orientation, language and recall are the focus of this standardised tool. An inability to answer less than 24 out of 30 of the questions is usually of concern. Even if the questions are answered correctly more sophisticated tests may be required. These further tests help identify specific problems in areas such as insight, comprehension and judgment.[3]

A screening tool for depression that the doctor may ask the patient to complete is the Geriatric Depression Scale (GDS, see Appendix IV). It is available in either a short or long form, and takes about ten to fifteen minutes to complete. It is a simple 'yes' or 'no' format.[4]

Medical history

The GP will ask for a comprehensive medical history, including:

- a list of past and present illnesses and operations;
- any current medication, both prescription and non-prescription;
- a drug and alcohol history;
- any incidence of depression;
- a history of any head trauma;
- a family history of Alzheimer's disease;
- the presence of potentially reversible syndromes that may present with dementia-like symptoms;
- a description of the onset and progression of cognitive deficits.

Physical examination

Physical examinations are routinely carried out by the doctor to assess general physical health and to identify and alleviate other treatable diseases such as Parkinson's disease or thyroid disorders. It will include a neurological examination.

Pathology tests

Some blood is taken for standard laboratory tests sometimes referred to as a dementia screen. The blood will be checked for vitamin deficiencies, chemical abnormalities, kidney and thyroid problems. Some doctors may go further and do a lumbar puncture to exclude meningitis or encephalitis, or ask for blood tests to rule out syphilis or AIDS depending on the history given. This last procedure is not routinely done.

Scans

An electroencephalogram (EEG) records the electrical activity of the brain much like an electrocardiogram (ECG) is performed to record the electrical activity of the heart. This procedure is done by attaching little wires to the surface of the scalp and is not invasive. It can be helpful in differentiating delirium from dementia, although it can appear normal when a person has dementia.

The patient will be referred for a computerised tomography (CT) scan (formerly known as a CAT or CT scan) or magnetic resonance imaging (MRI) to look for brain tumours, strokes or other dementias or brain conditions. Brain changes seen on the CT scan can indicate Alzheimer's disease, along with many other illnesses. A diagnosis is not made on the basis of the CT scan alone. An MRI provides a more detailed picture than a CT scan. The MRI provides more detailed anatomical information. For example, changes in a key memory centre of the brain called the entorhinal cortex, may be evident, especially if repeat MRI scans are performed 6 to 12 months apart.

As the Professor of Psychiatry at the New York University School of Medicine, Dr de Leon, said: 'The entorhinal cortex is the gateway to the hippocampus and is central to all memory functions in the brain. It is a memory distribution and processing centre and if its gate is broken, then new memories cannot be made and old memories cannot be retrieved.' Used routinely, MRI examination is not required for all people suspected of having dementia.

If a person is young or there is a strong family history of dementia, a position emission tomography (PET) scan will be performed where diagnosis is still unclear despite other investigations. It provides information much like the CT or MRI scan on the structure or skeleton of the brain. Based on his research Professor Gary Small, Director of the Centre on Ageing at the University of California, said: 'So you can see strokes, you can see brain shrinkage or atrophy, but it also provides much more information on brain function years before people might be at the age of risk when most people develop the disease.'[5]

Sometimes a diagnosis can occur when a person attends their doctor's surgery for a problem that they do not even consider to be a symptom of dementia. One extremely gifted, articulate 46-year-old woman had been having severe migraines that only went away on

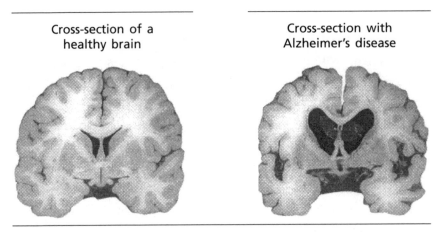

| Cross-section of a healthy brain | Cross-section with Alzheimer's disease |

Figure 3.1

The difference between a healthy brain and a diseased one.[6]

Sundays. Her local doctor, not suspecting Alzheimer's disease, had sent her for a routine CAT scan, a precautionary measure for persistent migraine. Her only reported problem was her headaches: fortunately, her dementing illness was diagnosed following a routine scan that revealed the true extent of her health issues.

> *When I had my first CAT scan I popped off from work for ten minutes and it was great to have a rest lying there having the scan done. When I pulled out the report, it said generalised atrophy; I could see the shrivelled walnut and the great hole in the middle of the brain where the inner hemispheric fissure is quite large. I thought, well, that is not very normal... and then I thought I would just carry on for the moment. Later I kept thinking that maybe this is not true. Maybe I have always had brain damage and I have just coped with it.*

Another example of a non-sequential set of circumstances in obtaining a diagnosis was reported by a carer's husband:

> *She had been to many different doctors, homeopaths, and a range of other types of people like chiropractors. She just felt sick and*

we thought it was a change of life, and she was depressed. She was seen as a hypochondriac. A new doctor referred her to a geriatrician. She was only forty-seven. She opened the referral letter and it said, 'I am really concerned that my patient has AD.' 'What is AD?' she asked. I said, 'Attention deficit, perhaps,' but it 'pinged' on me at the time.

Getting the results

It is advisable for a person with memory problems to take a friend or partner along when they get their results.

Having a support person is helpful as they will often remember or hear more clearly what is being said and can write it down. Often the person with Alzheimer's disease will have lots of questions to ask and will want information about the tests. They might want to request a copy of test results from their local doctor. The period between testing and learning the outcome is a difficult one, so the more support that is offered then, the less stressful the time will be for the individual. If no support person is available to attend the diagnostic interview, it is advisable that the person with memory problems takes along a notepad to write things down.

Well, he looked at the scans with his back to me and said, 'Oh, you have got Alzheimer's,' and it was a bolt out of the blue. I had seen the atrophy, but Alzheimer's had not crossed my mind. I knew that brain atrophy was serious, but I thought that maybe I had some condition that I had always lived with and I was obviously under too much stress for the amount of brain that I had. I really did not think that I had a medical condition. I said that I was too young. He replied, 'I have diagnosed people as young as thirty, and one lady was pregnant.'

This sufferer was also asked these questions:

Q. Do you think that some doctors have become desensitised, as a way of coping when giving people a dreadful diagnosis?

When there is a cancer they don't have to do it because...But that is because we have done our education about cancer, but I don't think that we have educated our medical practitioners sufficiently on what dementia is as a diagnosis. It is a psychosocial adaptation. With cancer the doctor can say, do x, y or z...

Q. Did you change doctors?

Yes, the second doctor was very different. When I asked the first doctor 'How long?', he said, 'About five years'. When I asked the second doctor the same question he said, 'Everyone is an individual,' and he would see me initially every three to six months and then every year and we would see how we went. He started me on an anti-dementia drug, which was very positive. He said, 'This drug might be able to help you, and certainly keep trying to do as much as you can. Keep up your driving and other social activities and interests.' He referred me to Oliver Sak's books...I now have read all of Sak's books. He takes me at face value.

There are many variances in how people are told about the diagnosis, and what information is offered at the point of diagnosis. Some people report being given information about where to get assistance, while others report that they were not given any information at all.

The doctors were very empathetic but neither suggested the Alzheimer's Association or support groups.

We went down to the snow. We were waiting for the results to come and when we got the letter saying, 'Yes, it was organic, they could not clearly diagnose Alzheimer's but it was dementia', a friend told us to start using a diary, to keep things stable, to keep things routine. I didn't believe it, it was absolutely devastating, and I believed he had a brain tumour. I don't remember what I was told.

On the first visit to the memory clinic we were told, 'We strongly suggest that you contact the Alzheimer's Association. I didn't know what that would do—I was too shocked...

I don't think that we did [contact the Association]. I have to say no to that initially, no to counselling.

Some people with a research background went directly to the Internet, some to local libraries or bookshops, while others phoned the Alzheimer's Association for support and information.

Informing the diagnosed person, family and friends

Whether to reveal to the sufferer, family members, work colleagues, friends, sports associates, religious groups and so on, the fact that a diagnosis of Alzheimer's disease has been made, is a difficult position. I have met hundreds of people with dementia and their families in my years of working as a counsellor. The two distinct approaches to this problem are further complicated by a multitude of family scenarios that are both unique and challenging.

One group is adamant about privacy and prefers to withhold the diagnosis for as long as possible, while the other group tells everybody as soon as possible. Part of the decision of whether or not to disclose is the concern that some negative impact might result: 'The rate of suicide among the elderly is high.'[7] A person with a long history of chronic depression needs to be assessed as to the appropriateness and the value of being told their diagnosis.

When a person learns that a member of their family has Alzheimer's disease, they may become overwhelmed by feelings of confusion, guilt and loneliness. Moreover, as they assume the role of caregiver they may feel hesitant to reveal the diagnosis to the person with the disease, to the rest of the family and to friends for fear their reactions will be difficult to manage.

Informing the sufferer

In deciding whether or not to tell the sufferer about the diagnosis, respect their right to know what's wrong but also be sensitive to their feelings and emotional state, medical condition and ability to remember, reason and make decisions.

Keep in mind that the person with Alzheimer's may suspect that something is wrong long before a doctor reaches a diagnosis. If no explanation is given they may assume the worst. On the other hand, if you discuss the problem with them, they may feel relieved to learn that they have a physical illness rather than a psychological one. Furthermore, the informed person may be able to participate in important medical, legal, financial and personal planning, depending on the progression of the disease symptoms.

Rely on professional experience. Consider informing the person about the diagnosis through a family conference, which may include the individual, other caregivers and a social worker. A physician who has experience working with cognitively impaired individuals could also be invited to attend.

Be sensitive to the sufferer's reactions. They may not be able to understand all that the diagnosis means, or they may deny the explanation. If this is the case, it's probably best to accept the reaction and avoid further detailed explanations of the disease. Reassure the person. Let them know that you'll provide ongoing help and support, and do all you can to make your lives together fulfilling.

When the time is right, provide the person with follow-up information that they would benefit from knowing, such as an explanation of symptoms and the importance of continued care. A carer may say,

'Mum, because of your memory and other problems, you may have to let people help you more than you have in the past.' Note that you don't have to use the phrase Alzheimer's disease if you think it might upset the person.

Treat the person as an adult, and don't downplay the disease. As the disease progresses, carers must remain open to the person's need to talk about the illness. The person may ask about activities such as working, driving or managing finances. They may want to express feelings of anger, frustration and disappointment. It is important to remain sensitive to non-verbal signs of sadness, anger or anxiety and respond with love and reassurance.

Informing family and friends

When informing family and friends be honest about the person's condition. You'll probably feel relieved after discussing the disease with other family members and close friends. Be sure to explain that Alzheimer's disease is a medical condition and not a psychological or emotional disorder or a contagious virus.

Provide others with adequate information on Alzheimer's disease, including a description of common symptoms. The more family and friends learn about the disease, the more comfortable they may feel around the person. Share educational material from the Alzheimer's Association, such as the brochure 'When the Diagnosis is Alzheimer's'. You may also want to invite close friends and family members to accompany you to a support group meeting sponsored by a local chapter of the Alzheimer's Association.

Don't leave yourself out of the conversation. Explain how the responsibility of caregiving has affected your life or may change your life in the future, so that others will have a better sense of how they can help. Ask for family support. Have several tasks in mind for people who say, 'Please let me know if there's anything I can do to help you.'

Involving others in caregiving will help them better understand your situation and why you've made certain decisions.

Ask people to come for short visits, but suggest they ring you first. Keep in mind that the person may become anxious if too many people visit at one time. In addition, recommend specific activities such as playing a simple game, taking a walk, or looking through a book of photographs with the person.[8]

People's social history and family experiences also affect whether or how they disclose a diagnosis. One delightful energetic eighty-year-old client explained her reasons for non-disclosure:

> *In my day we took a Christian perspective. Whatever cards life dealt you one just got on with it and managed—family matters stayed within the family. Everyone has some cross to bear and the diagnosis of dementia is our lot now. We have crossed many rivers in life and survived. The last thing that I need now is to have some neighbour come and tell me about my husband's behaviour. It is like when the children were at school and some mother would tell you about your child's behaviour before you either knew or had time to assess the situation. Back then I said, 'Just leave it with me, Mrs Smith, and I will take it from here, thank you very much.' Today this is still my partner and I will take it from here.*

This active client went to the Alzheimer's Association to ask about strategies that would help her to cope, as well as reading material she could digest in her own time. She was happy to have a private meeting at the Association, but was most unhappy about discussing her husband's condition with the other people in the village. Reprisal from other village inhabitants was immediately dismissed.

One young woman who tried to tell her husband's parents about his diagnosis got a less than supportive response:

> *Devastated, they did not believe it until they saw it in writing. I was horrified. I thought, 'I have known them for twenty-odd*

years. How could they think that I am making this all up?' I was given no support...I needed to cry, I needed someone to hold me and say that it was going to be okay. It was only when I went to work and burst into tears in front of my boss and said '[My husband]'s got Alzheimer's disease' that she got me the number of the Alzheimer's Association. That was the way I got any help after he [aged forty-seven] was diagnosed.

One lady experienced this response from her mother-in-law on disclosure:

I don't feel he has any support from his side of the family. Deep down she might think that it comes from her side of the family.

On the other hand, this family took a positive and collaborative approach:

The family all knew that he needed to have brain scans, and when we went to get the results, one of the children volunteered to come and take notes. After the meeting with the doctor she said, 'Would you like me to phone the rest of the family?' My sister said, 'Look, you have been dealing with this forgetfulness for some time now and you are very good at it. You know I am sure that you will be able to cope.'

One carer of a dementia sufferer said:

It's not like having someone diagnosed with heart disease. It is different. I just didn't want anyone to know. I did not want anyone to treat him differently, or treat me differently. We didn't tell the children, we agreed on that, we didn't tell many relatives. Our decision was based on our belief that they would treat him differently, like he was stupid. He had that idea from thirty years' experience dealing with people who are under some category of mental health. I wanted to protect him and I wanted to cover it up. I had lived with it in my family. I know about the stigma. Even though we are professionals.

Often the decision that is made about telling or not telling is the result of some lived experience. Some families share concerns and triumphs, while others share appropriate segments and keep quiet until they have had time to process the event and can make some sense of it all.

Some people are active in seeking information about the disease, while others do not want to know. There is no right way. What all people do want is to be understood and soothed. The fear of not being supported through this time is a good reason for non-disclosure. If, in the past, a person has experienced a lack of support for a major life event, they will hardly be likely to reach out for help at this time.

If you choose to disclose, be aware of the other person's perspective. They will generally ask a lot of questions that you may not yet know the answers to. If you are not emotionally robust enough to cope with the questions, and are concerned about inappropriate responses such as 'but s/he looks so normal' or 'do you really think that it is dementia?' it may be best to get more information and support before telling others. You will be coping with changes on many levels, and having to cope with non-helpful comments is best avoided until you feel more in control.

Innovative research is being undertaken by Dr Heather Wilkinson and Dr Murna Downs at the University of Stirling, Scotland, to study the effect on the person with dementia of being told the diagnosis.[9] The research is charting the experiences of thirty people who have been given the diagnosis the previous month. Patients will have the opportunity to discuss how the diagnosis was given and the immediate impact of the diagnosis, and will be given the opportunity to provide feedback on ways that this could be improved. A second interview will be conducted three months later to look at how the person has coped since the diagnosis, and how they feel about it now.

The right to know

Withholding the diagnosis of dementia from a patient was once regarded as best practice. It was in the interests of the person for a variety of reasons, ranging from the fear of their distress or suicide, and stigma about being different and therefore being treated as different. While there is still debate about whether or not to inform people about their diagnosis, there is a growing appreciation of the person's right to be told, especially now that people are being diagnosed a lot earlier. The potential benefit of being told the diagnosis is that it affords the person the right to make decisions and advanced plans: to address legal issues such as power of attorney options; to make a living will; or to move house if it is deemed necessary for future needs. The person with dementia can make positive contributions to these major decisions if they are diagnosed early and told the diagnosis.

Each person is an individual and each situation is unique. The decision to disclose or not to disclose needs careful thought and poses the question, 'Whose needs are being served best by this decision?' Non-disclosure can move carers, friends and family from a place of collaborative partnership to that of being a 'controller'.

Programs that are now being conducted for people in the early stage of dementia throughout Australia are based upon the person knowing the diagnosis. At this stage disclosure is viewed as being empowering for the person with dementia, certainly in terms of having the opportunity to discuss relevant issues such as employment, driving, feelings about increased dependency, not being asked about things, changes in their relationships with family and friends, and allowing the opportunity and time to discuss their issues. As one woman said: 'I weep for the lost opportunities for the future, no graduations, no marriages, no grandchildren—these sorts of things—[and] my daughter wept for losing her mum.' Sadly, at the time of diagnosis she was a 46-year-old scientist, a single parent with children not yet launched from home. When she rang the Alzheimer's Association they asked her if the sufferer was her father or her mother, and she said, 'Don't worry,' and put the phone down. She did not try again for another three years.

Available resources

Following a diagnosis of some form of dementia, people cope the best way that they know how. This is a very difficult time when emotions are running high and people are left feeling shocked, angry, stunned and totally out of control. This sense of powerlessness, injustice and rage is a very normal part of the grief reaction, as the ground has been taken from under their feet and it takes time for people to adjust to the diagnosis.

Some carers unfortunately do not move from this position of anger and rage at the unfairness of the situation and do not reach out for help for months or years after the diagnosis. They are incapable of seeking help because their level of grief is too overwhelming. This grief needs to be heard, supported and processed before they can take information on board or look at the situation through a different lens. What is paramount is that the person with dementia and the carer be advised that they can get professional support and process the grief issues rather than experiencing them alone. Knowing that there is help and support available is perhaps the greatest resource for the person with dementia and their carers.

Extensive scientific and psychosocial research conducted over the past ten years has resulted in early intervention programs and specialised assessment units designed specifically for people with dementia and their families.

Treatment options

Option A: Doctor and specialist management plan

The doctor is likely to refer the patient to a physician who specialises in dementia. This is especially true if the patient is young, as many of the assessment tools are geared towards people in older age groups. Often there is no evidence at this stage of brain abnormality, but the diagnostic tests will be repeated again in the next few months. People suffering from early Alzheimer's disease may show varying degrees of the early signs of the disease, such as memory loss, behavioural changes, changes in functionality along with mood changes or other physical problems such as headaches. A diagnosis may not be immediate, but the situation will be monitored regularly until the physician is confident the diagnostic criteria as set out in the DSM-IV (*Diagnostic and Statistical Manual of Mental Disorders* see Appendix II) have been met.[10] (The *Diagnostic and Statistical Manual of Mental Disorders* is a reference book published by the American Psychiatric Association, compiled by a group of international experts in different fields of mental health to formulate a consensus of diagnostic criteria. It is used by both clinicians and researchers, biological, psychodynamic, cognitive, behavioural, interpersonal and family/systems specialists, as well as physicians, psychiatrists, social workers, nurses and other health professionals.)

Once either a provisional diagnosis or a confirmed diagnosis is made, the patient and the carer are referred to the local doctor so that a management plan can be commenced. Ideally this management plan would include not only the current treatment for the person with dementia, but also the psychosocial needs of the carer and the family. The importance of a management plan that embraces the needs of the person with Alzheimer's disease, the carer and the family will be discussed in more depth in Parts three and four. If such a management plan is not forthcoming from the GP, a referral to the nearest Alzheimer's Association will provide the sufferers with ongoing information, support and advice. The development of a care plan gives the whole family something to focus on as the dementia progresses.

Option B: Specialised care centres

A person with Alzheimer's disease might choose to access one of the multidisciplinary Aged Care Assessment Teams (ACAT) that provide services for people over the age of sixty-five. Their primary role is to support the person with the illness or disability 'to maintain them in their home for as long as possible'. Recently, geriatric psychologists were appointed to ACATs in some areas to assess and treat the emotional and personal relationship issues involved with this older age group.

New specialist service centres have also been established as an extension of the ACATs. The Cognitive Dementia and Memory Services (CDAMS) are multidisciplinary specialised services that provide early diagnosis, specialised medical treatment, consultation, education, ongoing monitoring and support for people with cognitive deficits in all age groups. Services for people with dementia and their carers include:

- specific targeting of persons with the early stages of dementia;
- specialist skills in complex or unusual diagnoses of dementias;
- focus on informants/family/family involvement;
- access to drug trials for individuals with dementia;
- provision of tailored memory and cognitive strategies;
- provision of short-term counselling for family and individual problems;
- provision of regular reviews;
- twenty-four-hour help line services; and
- ongoing education and training.

In the past, dementia was viewed only as a medical condition. The new multidisciplinary approach provides assessment and referral to a wide range of services for those with cognitive problems, the purpose of which is to assist people with dementia to stay healthier longer, be better understood and to have a voice. The more supported and functional the family of the person with dementia is, the better the journey for the sufferer will be.

Specialist care centres provide a one-stop shop for people with dementia and their family. They work in conjunction with local doctors and provide a dual managed care approach. The regular monitoring of changes, either medically or psychosocially, are conducted in this team approach, which has the advantage of combining specialist and allied health staff to provide the person with dementia and their family with the best care and support. These services are available to all those who are concerned about memory problems.

Option C: Rejection of specialist help

Professional staff involved in the support of people with dementia can include physicians, geriatricians, neuropsychologists, psychologists, community nurses, speech pathologists, occupational therapists, counsellors, social workers and educators.[11] If people do not seek a diagnosis, then they and their family may be excluded from the wide range of treatments and services available. The avoidance of making early decisions about medical management, financial planning and the execution of legal matters will impact severely on the management of the illness later. It should also be remembered that there are now new therapies available that can slow down the progress of Alzheimer's disease.

It cannot be stressed strongly enough that by far the most important thing that people need at this time is emotional support—to be heard, to be held and to be valued through the trauma they are experiencing. This is a time of grief and of multiple losses; each individual will have different experiences including loss of the known self, loss of the person as you have known them, loss of dreams, hopes and wishes, loss of a planned future, loss of self-esteem and/or self-confidence. It is a time of adaptation and challenges.

When people are ready they can access information from the Alzheimer's Association about dementia via:

- a national helpline in the UK 0845 300 0336;
- a national helpline in Ireland 1800 341 341;
- a professional counselling service that is private and confidential;
- a support group for people with early stage dementia;
- a dementia-specific library;
- the Internet;
- the Living with Memory Loss Program;
- membership benefits;
- family education seminars with dementia-specific topics; and
- workshops and conferences about dementia.

People can be advised, supported and gently directed, but it is only when they are ready that they will seek help. Unfortunately, most of the people seen at the Alzheimer's Association have been battling for a long time with minimal support or information before a crisis situation, a loss of their own health or a painful family breakdown causes them to seek support.

Dementia is now openly tabled as a world health problem that affects one in twenty people over the age of sixty-five. People with dementia need access to information, a coordinated medical approach and a family with the functionality to absorb the person with dementia in the early stages. As with any other chronic illness, there is a new language to learn, a new set of strategies to be adopted, a new way of living that is manageable. There are many resources available. The first step is to just pick up the phone and ask your questions.

4 Behavioural changes

ALTHOUGH THE BRAIN IS THE CENTRE OF EXISTENCE, PEOPLE USUALLY do not take much notice of it until there are changes or problems that affect them. The brain is a very emotionally charged point of reference with both negative and positive connotations. For the entirety of your life its functionality is a marker upon which you gauge competence.

Once a child's gender is established the scene is set for a range of predictable gender-based comments in the first few years of life, for example, 'Isn't she cute?' or 'That's my boy!'. All goes well unless the child fails to develop normally or achieve some milestone. Eventually, investigations occur that will involve some aspect of the brain.

A person's life is 'normal' until there occurs microscopic changes in the brain that initially may not even be detected in a brain scan. The first signs are often lapses of memory.

Dementia is a cluster of symptoms that are associated with different underlying diseases. It is not a normal part of ageing and it will affect different aspects of a person's thinking, behaviour, mood and personality. There is generally no pain, fever or wounds. There is no bacterial or causative virus to be identified, investigated or understood. The person with dementia is alert, fully conscious and does all the normal activities of daily living: showering, dressing, driving a car, watching TV, mowing the lawn and playing with the dog. He/she may still be employed. It is often only memory or speech changes, or slight changes in behaviour, that are different.

Carers often doubt the reality of the problem even after the diagnosis or provisional diagnosis has been made. Carers keep looking for the changes. Some days they can't see anything, which is understandable as brain changes are not as immediately obvious as in a physical illness. Even in the middle and later stages of the disease some carers will still try to communicate in the same way that they have for the past twenty or fifty years, usually because they have either not been able to accept that the person's brain changes will prevent them from remaining the same, or they may have never been told what to expect. Regardless of whether they are or are not diagnosed with dementia, some people will not begin to understand the process and therefore have problems trying to learn to live with what they don't understand.

The underpinning issue is the unseen damage to the nerve cells in the brain that control behaviour in the early, moderate and later stages of dementia. We do not expect a person with a broken leg to be able to dance, but when people are diagnosed with dementia we expect the person to behave as they have always done. There is often some part of us that has great difficulty accepting what we cannot see. One child describes her experience of her father's dementia:

> *Well, sometimes I'd tell one of my friends and she tried to understand, but one would really not understand if they were not living with it. They kind of want proof about it, because they can't see it. He is standing there and physically, he looks normal. If he had had his appendix out there would be a scar.*

Having some basic understanding about the brain and how it affects behaviour assists in making some sense of the difficulties people with dementia experience throughout their day. Allowing changed behaviour to become the focus of attention creates distress and frustration to both the person with the disease and the family carer.

It makes a lot more sense to work smarter than harder—we would never dream of taking someone's spectacles and expecting them to read small print from three metres away. If you find yourself asking, 'Why did you...?', remind yourself always that the person with dementia does not know! Changed behaviour occurs because of damage to the brain cells; it has nothing to do with the person choosing to be difficult.

Degenerative brain diseases affect at least two people—those who are battling with the losses, and those who love and care for them. The information in this chapter will hopefully explain what can be happening between the brain and the person's behaviour. If you want more specific information, your doctor, neurologist or gerontologist will be more than happy to supply this.

The brain

The function of the human brain is unparalleled by anything in the world. It is an incredibly complex organ composed of billions of microscopic neurons or brain cells. Daily activities like walking, talking, learning, remembering, working, creating, occur when brain cells communicate with each other. If the mechanism of communication between the cells is interrupted or damaged by disease, such as a dementing illness, the brain is unable to do its job in some areas. This is observable through changes in a person's memory, thinking or behaviour.

Brain surface

The outer surface of the brain is known as the *cerebral cortex*. The surface or *cortex* of the brain consists of many nooks and crannies resembling mountain ranges on a map.

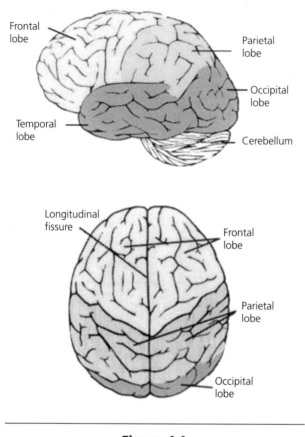

Figure 4.1
The parts of the brain.[1]

The cortex is divided into two halves called *hemispheres*. The left hemisphere is often called the dominant side as it is the language centre for most people. The right hemisphere is commonly referred to as the non-dominant side of the brain and is spatially oriented.[2] The structure of the cortex is extremely complicated and it is here that the high-level functions associated with the mind are implemented.

Both of the hemispheres are further divided into four lobes, and each lobe performs specific functions depending on which side of the brain they are on. Table 4.1 (see page 55) provides a summary

Table 4.1

A summary of behavioural effects[3]

Effect on behaviour	Examples	Area of the brain affected
Unable to remember words that are read, seen or heard (memory)	• recent memories quickly lost • forget people and events	Temporal lobe (memory centre)
Unable to use language (speech, writing and reading) to communicate (language expression)	Difficulty: • saying precisely what they want to say • naming common objects • understanding what is said to them	Parietal lobe (left side) (analytical and logical centre) (right changes to left)
Unable to locate position of the person or objects in space (spatial awareness)	Difficulty: • knowing how to get somewhere • locating the car in the car park	Parietal lobe (right side) (analytical and logical centre) (left changes to right)
Unable to carry out planned or learned patterns of movement (apraxia)	Difficulty: • putting clothes on in correct order • using appliances such as stove, car • putting tablecloth on the table	Parietal lobe (both sides)
Unable to recognise things (agnosia)	Unable to recognise: • family member(s) • objects such as knives, forks • surroundings such as their house	Parietal lobe (both lobes)
Unable to plan or organise (insight)	• shops without money • don't dress appropriately but believe they have • not aware of the state of tidiness of the house	Front lobe (executive centre)

Effect on behaviour	Examples	Area of the brain affected
Unable to start an action (initiation)	Appear: • apathetic • unmotivated	Frontal lobe (executive centre)
Unable to stop once starting or saying something (perseveration)	Repeat: • questions • statements • actions	Frontal lobe (executive centre)
Unable to keep on track and control social behaviour (regulation)	• easily distracted • wanders • talks over others	Frontal lobe (executive centre)
Unable to correct behaviours, emotions and memories (connection)	• angry responses • accusations of stealing	Limbic region (connecting centre)

of the functions that may be affected when a particular part of the brain degenerates.

Frontal lobes: The executive centre

The frontal lobes are critical for learning and remembering new verbal information. They govern motor functions, emotions, speech, personality, social behaviour and inhibitions. They solve problems with planning and organising, remembering people and events, and are closely linked with making decisions and judgments.

When affected, they may interfere with a person's ability to see things as they really are.

For example, a person with dementia might:

• see the world as 'just rosy' while family carers are riddled with stress;

- have personality changes—become noisy and boisterous when pre-viously they may have been shy and retiring;
- say or do inappropriate things in mixed company, and see no prob-lem with their behaviour;
- laugh at their own jokes, and lose sensitivity to other people or the environment;
- forget to take money when shopping;
- lose insight about their dress sense and state of tidiness in the house or office;
- repeat questions, statements and actions;
- be easily distracted—they may talk over others.

Parietal lobes: The language expression and spatial centre

The parietal lobes are responsible for our sensory functions like touch and spatial senses, our ability to do mathematics and to know where we are in time, space and position.

When affected, the person may experience difficulty with:

- the judgment of distances;
- knowing how to get to a place;
- finding their car in a parking station;
- putting on clothes—for example, they may put swimwear over their street clothes, or be unable to do up buttons;
- recognising family members, familiar objects and surroundings;
- saying exactly what they want to say; and
- understanding what is actually said to them.

Temporal lobes: The memory centre

The temporal lobes involve hallucinations, memory, vision, hearing and verbal understanding, as well as memory of emotions such as happiness, jealousy, anger or fear.

With a dementing illness different areas are affected unevenly and a person will be able to do some things and not others. Some parts of the brain may be damaged, while other areas may not be damaged at all. The focus of care and functionality should centre on the non-affected areas, which reinforces the need for cognitive testing to clarify what the problem is and where a person's strengths remain. The role of the carer is to accentuate the positive aspects and work around the affected parts. Understanding is the key to moving from a position of adversity to one of mastery.

5 Drug treatments

IT WAS ONCE UNCOMMON FOR DEMENTIA TO ACTUALLY BE NAMED, which saved many health professionals from having to deal with the lack of treatment options or from having to tell the family or patient that nothing could be done. If a diagnosis was made, the issue was often dismissed as being a natural part of ageing. It is very difficult not to have any solutions in a solution-focused world. Gypsies and horse doctors knew the benefit of giving people 'something', even if it did not work. The value of offering a potion or a cure-all has served most people well—except those people with dementia.

When in the 1970s it was discovered that an essential neurotransmitter that affects nerve endings in the brain was deficient in people with Alzheimer's disease, major drug companies sponsored clinical trials into new treatments for dementia. But these drugs are not cures. Hope in the form of a future cure was what the world had been waiting for. Until a few years ago, no suitable drugs were available. In 2001, Harvard University neurologist Dr Dennis Seloke, in an interview for *Time* magazine, stated that: 'we will shortly have on hand, not one, but several drugs capable of slowing down or even halting the progressions of the disease...even better is the diagnostic ability to diagnose patients a lot earlier so that they can receive treatment before their brains fade.'[1]

Acetylcholine—the missing link

At the Albert Einstein School of Medicine in the early 1970s, Dr Peter Davies discovered that a particular enzyme was depleted in the brains of people with Alzheimer's disease.[2] This enzyme, cholineacetyltransferase, helps the body's chemical reactions work and is essential for the production of a brain messenger molecule called acetylcholine. A message (electrical signal) is sent along the nerve fibre when nerve cells want to communicate with other nerve cells. The electrical signal causes acetylcholine to be released. It floats across the gap between the cells and causes the waiting nerve cell to start up another electrical signal, which travels to the end of its fibres, releases other messages to float across the gaps and make the connections. Acetylcholine is the enzyme responsible for this activity, and chlorine- acetyltransferase makes acetylcholine.

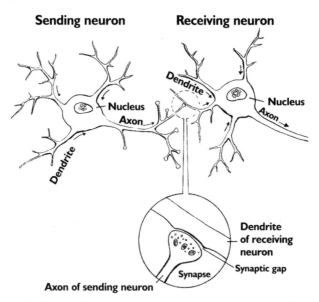

The lower enlarged area shows the synapse in some detail,
while the upper area shows how it fits into the overall neuronal structure.

Figure 5.1

Basic neuronal structure.[3]

In Alzheimer's disease it is thought there are chemical changes in the brain that lower the level of the neurotransmitting acetylcholine. Insufficient levels of acetylcholine interfere with the brain's cholinergic system, most likely leading to cognitive and memory impairment. Following the discovery of the reduced amounts of acetylcholine in the brains of people with Alzheimer's disease, drug research focused on ways to either increase the amount of the neurotransmitter in the brain or to copy the process that naturally occurs in non-diseased brains.

The first breakthrough

In 1993 the United States approved the first treatment for Alzheimer's disease: a drug called tacrine (brand name Cognex). Studies of this drug show that some people found it helpful but others did not respond, that it could cause liver damage if given to some patients in high doses, and that it required regular blood tests to monitor liver function. In the end the side effects outweighed the benefits and it has been withdrawn.

Improvements in anticholinesterase treatments

Anticholinesterase drugs are now available for people in the early to moderate stages of dementia. Three such drugs currently available are donezepil (Aricept), rivastigmine (Exelon) and galantamine (Reminyl) (see page 65).

There are many other acetylcholinesterase inhibitors being tested. In particular, galantamine, marketed as Reminyl. This class of drug offers people an opportunity to delay the onset of the symptoms and, while not a cure, the delay of the symptoms offers hope—people are very grateful for having more time to psychologically adjust to their condition.

It has been reported that the improvements in cognition that result from taking anticholinesterase drugs have been accompanied by changes in behaviour and mood. The major changes reported were reduction of anxiety and distress and the restoration and maintenance of confidence for the person with dementia. Any improvement in mood has a positive impact on the person with dementia, the family carer and the family itself.

Researchers at the Alzheimer's Disease Society in London have proposed a study on the quality of life for persons with dementia and their carers as an urgent priority.[4] The research report will highlight the realistic expectations that anticholinesterase drugs offer for the person with dementia and their carers. The researchers know that the possibility of holding back the tide has given sufferers more confidence, and hope that this will convince the many specialists who are not persuaded of the value of treatment regimes to begin offering them immediately.[5]

Commencing treatment

This requires thorough assessment, and preferably specialist confirmation of the diagnosis. It is important that there is a realistic understanding of the potential benefits of these treatments and that consent is obtained. A Mini Mental State Examination (MMSE, see page 33 and Appendix III) is administered before commencing treatment with the patient having a mild to moderate dementia (which usually rates between 10 and 25 on the MMSE scale).[6] The test is repeated at regular intervals to see if the drug is working.

Monitoring progress

A family member should monitor compliance, note changes in mood and behaviour and observe any adverse side effects. Both the patient and the carer should be able to recognise the usefulness of the treatment, and understand that the treatment may cease if there are adverse side effects, poor compliance, or a deterioration of the patient's condition.

A recent publication stated that the new anti-Alzheimer's drugs were recommended for use by people in the early stages of dementia who 'had symptom duration of six months or more', this being the same criteria used in the World Health Organisation's tenth revision of the International Classification of Diseases (Chapter V). However, some patients wish to commence taking the anti-dementia drugs earlier to improve their chances of delaying the symptoms.[7]

Anti-dementia drug treatments

This following discussion provides information about how these drug treatments work, who might benefit and what questions people with dementia, their families and carers should ask their doctor before being prescribed any of the drugs.

Acetylcholinesterase inhibitor drugs

How these drugs work

Drugs known as acetylcholinesterase inhibitors work on one part of the system of chemical messages by preventing or inhibiting acetylcholinesterase from working. This means that there is more acetylcholine, the chemical messenger, available and there is more chance of the acetylcholine being passed on to the next nerve cell and transmitting the message.

The increased communication between nerve cells may temporarily improve or stabilise the symptoms of the disease. However, it is unlikely that a defect in acetylcholine levels is the only or indeed the main deficit in Alzheimer's disease. The use of acetylcholinesterase inhibitors is only one possible pharmaceutical approach to treating the symptoms.

The effect of these treatments

The effect of acetylcholinesterase inhibitor drugs varies. About one in three will not notice any effect, while about a third find that their condition improves slightly and a third stabilise, when they would have expected to become gradually less able. The areas that some people with Alzheimer's disease may find improvement in are the ability to think clearly, function in daily activities such as managing the bank account, talking and dressing, and a reduction in behavioural changes such as apathy, hallucinations and delusions.

Trials indicate that the drugs delay the progression of symptoms for about nine to twelve months on average. This does not mean that the drugs should be stopped after nine to twelve months—otherwise, the delay in the progression of symptoms will be lost. Some people with dementia report benefits for longer periods.

Who will benefit?

Acetylcholinesterase inhibitor drugs are approved for use by people with mild to moderate Alzheimer's disease. There is some evidence that the earlier the drugs are started the better. Clinical trials for Exelon, Aricept and Reminyl for the treatment of severe Alzheimer's disease are currently underway. People who have a less common form of dementia called Lewy Body or diffuse Lewy Body disease have also been shown to benefit, and there is emerging evidence that people with both vascular dementia and Alzheimer's disease may also benefit.

Clinical trials showed no difference in the effectiveness of the drugs relating to age, sex or ethnic origin.

The drugs treat the symptoms of Alzheimer's disease only and should not be considered a cure—there is no evidence that they can halt or reverse the process of cell damage that causes the disease. It is also important to realise that these drugs will not help everyone who tries them.

The following information concerns those acetylcholinesterase inhibitor drugs that are registered in Australia, New Zealand, USA, UK and other countries around the world. They can only be prescribed by a medical practitioner. Comprehensive product information should be consulted before taking these medications.

Donezepil hydrochloride—Aricept
A piperidine-based selective acetylcholinesterase inhibitor which is highly selective for acetylcholinesterase in the central nervous system. It significantly inhibits brain cholinesterase.

Rivastigmine—Exelon
Rivastigmine is a cholinesterase inhibitor that inhibits both acetylcholinesterase and butyrylcholinesterase, which may theoretically be advantageous, as central nervous system butyrylcholinesterase levels are raised in individuals with Alzheimer's disease.

Galantamine—Reminyl
Galantamine is a selective, competitive and reversible acetylcholinesterase inhibitor with a dual mode of action through allosteric modification of presynaptic nicotinic receptors.[8]

The side effects from taking these drugs are more common at the beginning, but they often settle down with time. The most likely side effects are diarrhoea, nausea, vomiting, muscle cramps, insomnia, fatigue and loss of appetite. Other reported side effects include dizziness and nightmares. If the dose is increased gradually the likelihood of side effects is less. Caution is required in people with a history of peptic ulcer, asthma or abnormally slow heart rates.

Tacrine Hydrochloride—Cognex
The name used for marketing tacrine hydrochloride is Cognex. It has a relatively high rate of side effects—in particular on the liver—and has been superseded by newer compounds.

How to get treatment

It is important that people obtain a proper diagnosis and assessment to establish whether they have Alzheimer's disease or another form of dementia, and whether they are in the early or moderate stage of the illness. A specialist such as a neurologist, psychogeriatrician, geriatrician or psychiatrist should make the assessment and prescribe the drugs. A general practitioner can also prescribe them.

Whenever a person begins taking a new drug the doctor, patient and family members should discuss the potential side effects and how the drug may interact with any other medicines being taken. The questions to ask your doctor about any drug being prescribed should include:

- What are the potential benefits of taking the drug?
- How long should the person take the drug before a response can be detected?
- How often is it administered to people with Alzheimer's disease?
- What should I do if the person misses taking a dose?
- What are the known side effects?
- If the person has side effects, should I reduce the dosage or should I stop the drug immediately?
- If the drug is stopped suddenly, what happens to the patient?
- What drugs (prescription and over-the-counter) might interact with the medication?
- How might this drug affect other medical conditions?
- What changes in the patient's condition should be reported immediately?

- How often will the person need to visit the doctor who prescribed the drug?
- When should the medication be ceased?

The only way to see if new drug treatments are working is to regularly monitor the person with dementia, for example by cognitive testing using the Mini Mental State Examination (MMSE).

Clinic drug trials and other studies

The media often alert people to potential new drug treatments in the embryonic stages. However, it may be years before people are asked to participate in drug trials after a media release and then years again before large scale trials are completed. A recent report on the front page of the Melbourne *Age* captured this succinctly when reporting about a drug being tested: 'PBT–1 is the culmination of more than $10 million in development costs and over a decade of research. It will be at least four years until the drug being tested becomes publicly available.'[9]

People in the early to moderate stages of dementia are the most likely research candidates, as people in the later stages probably have irreversible brain damage. Any person who does volunteer for such programs will benefit not only themselves from the scientific research, but will also assist those who will be diagnosed in the future. It is important that people who do participate in trials don't hold unrealistic expectations of a cure. Most of the pharmaceutical drugs available now for treating dementia do not purport to be a cure; rather, researchers advocate that they have made an 'exciting advance…and are looking for drugs that can be effective to at least partially modify the course of the illness'.[10]

Families and research subjects need to carefully consider many issues prior to embarking on drug trials. People contemplating participation in drug research should ask about:

- the purpose of the study;
- how the study will be conducted;
- the method of administration of the drug;
- the size and safety of the dosage given;
- the potential side effects;
- the definite side effects;
- the consent of the subject;
- any travel and accommodation expenses;
- the credentials of researchers; and
- support and attitude towards subjects and family carers.[11]

The uptake of any drug will be different for each individual and may be affected by, for example, other diseases co-existing with dementia, the degree of dementia, the age of onset of dementia, infections, incorrect diagnosis of dementia and changes in mood and behaviours.

Alternative treatments

The anti-dementia drug treatments increase the level of acetylcholine and help the brain to maintain its level of functioning for longer. This, however, does not stop the loss of nerve cells so many people often use other therapies as well.

While alternative therapies will not cure people with dementia, they can have a positive influence on a person's quality of life.

People in the early stages of dementia often lack the ability to instigate or follow through with occupational or recreational activities. Having the opportunity to engage in alternative therapies as an enjoyable social activity can be advantageous, although it is imperative that the person with dementia is given the choice of whether or not to participate.

The current plethora of therapies used in the care of people with dementia includes music therapy, art therapy, reminiscence therapy, validation therapy, reality orientation therapy, massage, aromatherapy, herbal medicine, and acupuncture. People use these remedies in conjunction with medical treatments.

There are controlled studies that support the use of alternative therapies for the person with dementia. The fact that they make people feel better is perhaps as good as it gets. The downside is that people may create financial problems for themselves and the family as they pursue a quick fix solution for this problem. Generally, advertisers of such new treatments do not have to bear the scrutiny to which the medical profession is subjected. It would be wise to hasten gently and weigh up both the positive experience and the costs of alternative therapies.

Recent studies suggest that anti-oxidants might help to slow down the progress of dementia. Working in this field, Christine Bryden (formerly Boden), herself diagnosed with dementia, notes that there are many hypotheses about the value of anti-oxidants, but offers her current regime to people with dementia: vitamin E (2000 IU), vitamin C (1 g) and lecithin (2400 mg) per day. She also states: 'It does seem as if they have helped a bit in making me feel a little less foggy in the head...But it is really hard to know for sure.'[12]

There is also some evidence that suggests that the daily use of non-steroidal anti-inflammatory drugs (NSAIDS) may be of some use. Use as a treatment for Alzheimer's disease failed to show benefit over a placebo. NSAIDS may yet be shown to help delay or prevent the onset of the disease. There are risks with taking NSAIDS, namely adverse effects on the stomach.

Evidence now exists which supports the notion that women who use hormone replacement therapy (HRT) are less likely to develop dementia than those who do not use it. HRT failed in trials as a treatment but may yet be shown to be useful in prevention.[13]

Ginkgo biloba, a popular herb used by people with dementia, certainly causes no harm except it may exacerbate a bleeding tendency and may be found to retard the progression of the disease. The leaves of this plant have been used since the Ming Dynasty to help brain function and to relieve the symptoms of asthma and coughing. Ginkgo biloba has anti-oxidant, anti-platelet aggregator (blood thinner) and other properties. Small research studies conducted in Europe showed improvements in people with mild to moderate dementia, although the researchers were unable to produce conclusive evidence.[14]

Despite the considerable amount of research with the general public, there is no empirical evidence that alternative therapies have a curative component for people with dementia. For the purposes of clarity, the value of these therapies is best categorised under the heading of caring.

part two

Living with dementia

6 A rite of passage

A RITE IS A SOLEMN ACT CUSTOMARY IN RELIGIOUS SETTINGS, WHEREAS a rite of passage is a ceremony marking an individual's advance through life such as adulthood, marriage, birth, death.

The advantage of celebrating a rite of passage is that everyone understands why they are there and what they are celebrating, but what about other happenings in a person's life that have no rite or ritual associated?

How different would it be if you could, in some way, acknowledge the downside of life such as the loss of a limb, a child with a disability, retrenchment, financial losses, loss of health, loss of capacity to function in the same way as before, or loss of a relationship.

There are many days commemorated through some form of ritual, even if it is only the purchase of a red plastic nose to adorn the front of a commercial van. How different is it for people whose losses are publicly recognised to those who aren't?

Grief and disenfranchised loss

No ritual or rite of passage occurs to mark the changes that occur when a family member is diagnosed with dementia. In most cases following the diagnosis people are often left to their own devices to cope with the major adaptations required as best they can. People who have worked in jobs for twenty years may, following the diagnosis of dementia, walk out of the door and not return—they virtually cease to exist. There is no congratulatory card for early and untimely retirement. People do not know what to do, or how to react other than to say to a work colleague, 'Isn't it awful about Harry, Joe or Pam?'. There is no social construction to acknowledge this traumatic event, that is, the diagnosis of a dementing illness, because the event is often totally ignored.

Professor Kenneth Doka, a gerontologist and counsellor from Canada, states: 'There are circumstances in which a person experiences a sense of loss but does not have a socially recognised right, role, or capacity to grieve. In these cases, the grief is disenfranchised.'[1] Disenfranchised grief may also be experienced as a result of suicide, abortion, the death of a lover, a developmental disability or AIDS.

People with dementia almost always experience the loss of their capacity to function independently, to live their life by choice. When the nerve endings in the brain slowly start to die, it is not socially recognised as 'loss'.

When one 57-year-old man received the diagnosis of dementia, he had never heard of the word. He said:

> I feel claustrophobic, I could kick it, they keep you in the dark and feed you bullshit. I call this a shit of a frustrating disease. My company went bust, I lost the lot. I no longer have faith. When I received the diagnosis I felt there was nothing that I could do except get my shotgun out and use it.

Receiving a diagnosis of dementia can be catastrophic for many people when they are not in the accepted age range. In the above-mentioned person's history his diagnosis was compounded by severe financial losses. His suffering does not have a social definition for grieving, as it is not as yet codified by mainstream society.

Attachments to one's health, the future, the proceeds of a working life and investments, 'what might have been', are all shattered. One could hypothesise that the billions spent annually on anti-stress and anti-depressant medication is only chemical management for many losses that go unrecognised, and it is often falsely assumed that people can just build a bridge and get on with it. The question remains, how?

Out of sight out of mind?

Whole families or family carers can suffer from a psychosocial death wherein the persona of someone changes significantly through 'mental illness or organic brain syndromes (dementia)...[so that] significant others perceive the person as he or she previously existed, and as now dead'.[2] This can be witnessed when a person is diagnosed with a dementing illness and work colleagues cease to visit or phone the home, and one by one social contacts diminish. This profound sense of loss that spouses and others may experience cannot be publicly acknowledged as the person is still alive. There is no social recognition of the loss of the relationship as it was known, the loss of hopes, dreams and future plans. 'The emotional reactions can be complicated when grief is disenfranchised ... It can intensify the feeling of anger, guilt or powerlessness'.[3]

I support the growing notion that regardless of the age of people at the time of diagnosis of dementia, the process of loss and grief needs to be acknowledged as a legitimate part of their experience. Whatever the spiritual beliefs of the individual, the spirit, the essential being, does not age. If these two issues, the rite of passage into dementia and disenfranchised grief, were more appropriately addressed, then some of the causes of depression in our society could surely be reduced.

An international emblem depicting dementia could be developed that could be worn on a set day to acknowledge the loss of the person as they had been known, as other organisations do. This public acknowledgement of a shared silent loss while the person is still alive would also acknowledge the people in hostels and nursing homes who are no longer visited by, or of interest to, families. These people do exist and, while their care is undertaken by non-family members, their existence as part of the human race could be saluted.

Society has changed

If you are middle-aged, you would by now have survived many of the vicissitudes of life common to most people in some form or other: school, work, housing, children, marriage, redundancy, financial instability, career changes and the making or losing of friends, parents or children.

You would have seen the legalisation of many things that were forbidden in your youth, from homosexuality to unrestricted drinking and gambling. Conversely, many other events that were once common have now been restricted; for example, smoking, drink driving, discrimination against women, racial vilification, restrictive industrial practices and environmental pollution.

Families have changed

Families no longer just consist of dad, mum and from two to four children. Today families may be reconstituted every seven years, with a change in partners, in-laws and children, and additional children with each new relationship.

This macro view of changes to the family often does not include older people or grandparents from both sets of parents, and the care that they may require in the future. Nor does it include people in their forties, fifties and sixties who are diagnosed with a debilitating illness and still have children living at home. Yet it is the family in whatever form that has a significant role in the care of a person with a dementing illness.

With so many changes to the fundamental structure of family life, it is no wonder that people are in need of support when a member of the family suffers from some kind of dementia. Family cohesion will be challenged and tested as the family adjusts to the changes that have been imposed upon it. Alternatively, pre-existing conflicts will be exacerbated as the family structure begins to change soon after the diagnosis of a dementing illness occurs.

Carer profile

The average age of a carer is forty-five to sixty-five years of age and is most likely female; in fact, 'daughters outnumber sons as primary caregivers 4 to 1'.[4] Female carers are much more likely to be in the workforce than were their counterparts in the past, so these 'women in the middle' are faced with the unprecedented challenge of balancing the needs of several generations that may or may not live in the same household or regional area.

Social acceptance of mental health

Breakthroughs in science and technology have been exponential. People can universally access information, credit, goods and services, vice and pleasure while sitting in their own homes. It is now possible to have their organs transplanted, bits of silicone inserted into strategic places in their bodies and live to tell the story. Physical illness and treatment regimes are a multimillion dollar business and can be seen on TV or the Internet at the flick of a switch. It is the 'get it out on the table and let's talk about it era'. Sex, drugs, abuse, death, genetic engineering, genocide, suicide and mental health: these topics are now acceptable for social discourse, policy-making and sometimes even collective action.

While our external appearances and environment may have changed dramatically, it seems that despite all our sophisticated talk our inner lives have been unable to keep up with all these changes. We can still feel just as disappointed, hurt, fearful, depressed and ashamed as in the past.

Shame and depression

Many of the people who were interviewed for this book kept secret the diagnosis of dementia, the major reason for secrecy being that they were afraid that they or the person with dementia would be treated differently. This was the last thing they needed at the time. Depression, including suicidal thoughts, is the earliest and most prevalent reaction to dementia. It has been found that 30 per cent of newly diagnosed people are clinically depressed, and 63 per cent of people self-diagnose as depressed.[5]

Graham Burrows, Professor of Psychiatry at the University of Melbourne, describes 'our quiet crisis' and says that 'the most stressful thing in life is between our ears', or in the realms of mental functioning.[6] Depression will be the second highest leading cause of disability by 2020. In 1998 Australians spent $4 billion on legal drugs to counter stress and about $186 million on anti-depressants alone.[7]

So what is going wrong? We have more material assets than ever before, yet an epidemic of depression. Many people with depression or stress-related mental health issues might spend years on anti-depressant medication, as dementia and depression in the early stages can look similar. Personal strengths and a sense of wellbeing can become increasingly reduced in people with dementia, to compensate for the changes they are feeling and noticing but do not understand. As the wife of a 47-year-old dementia patient sadly reflected:

> *They said at his work that he needed to go and see 'someone'. He went to his doctor and he was diagnosed with depression and they put him off work for a couple of weeks. He was then sent to a psychiatrist, who treated him for depression for a considerable length of time.*

Many people with dementia can develop depression, anxiety or paranoia, symptoms that can be one of the first changes experienced or noticed by others. Science and technology have so far been unable to protect us from the reality that we will eventually age and lose the mastery of our environment. In terms of people with dementia or brain problems, we still have a lot to learn.

Living alone

Whereas people with dementia were once put into psychiatric hospitals, now with the de-institutionalisation of mental health, people with dementia are no longer shut up as if they did not exist. They are a part of society and require a place that is meaningful and purposeful, both for themselves and for those that offer care.

Dementia is no longer something experienced by one's aged parents and absorbed by the care of extended families. Having an aged parent live permanently in the family home is a thing of the past, as research reveals that older people would prefer to live alone than share with their children: 'Elderly people desire more than anything the preservation of their independence, they desire "intimacy at a distance" with their relatives...two or three generational households require considerable adjustment on the part of the elderly.'[8]

A lot of people over the age of forty now live alone (either by choice or circumstance) or are in de facto relationships. Many of them do not have the extended family system to offer support. Retirees may make financial decisions to move to coastal areas while their children remain closer to work in another city, state or country. This geographical distancing makes care options difficult, further isolating those with dementia and their carers from family support.

Moving into the mainstream

There is no quick fix for the social and demographic issues, however, improvement has already occurred in response to other major traumatic life events. Twenty years ago when a child died during or after birth, it was often whisked away never to be seen. Thankfully today all that has changed. Grief and bereavement have become topics of workshops and seminars. Books have been written, television interviews have been conducted and radio programs have moved grief from the hub of the family to mainstream consciousness. The result is that there is now a rite of passage, offered to people to mark the place in their lives where they have suffered, a place that gives some meaning to the loss on a deeper level.

The future

It is unprecedented that so many people are living beyond the age of sixty. Between 1990 and 2010, the number of dementia cases in more developed countries is projected to increase from 7.4 million to 10.2 million (a 37 per cent increase).

As dementia increases exponentially with age, some assistance is required for people who will need to manage at home for between three and five years before community services will be required by them. It is not just the physical health problems that wear out carers at this stage; it is often also the changed relationship with the sufferer and the difficulties in understanding the nature and progress of dementia.

Information, support and education from shared experiences are needed to create more understanding and to ensure a less traumatic journey for all concerned.

7 Beyond the patient: partners, family and friends

AS PREVIOUSLY STATED, LONG BEFORE THERE IS A DIAGNOSIS OF a dementing illness there have been changes in the family that have been noticed, denied or worried about, depending on the type of relationship that a person has with the patient. If the relationship holds great significance, the concerns about what may be likely to occur can cause anxiety and stress. If the relationship is not as significant there will be a lesser impact. This chapter is about carers who have meaningful attachments to the person with the dementing illness who have experienced the changes over the preceding years and have expressed concerns for the patient and worries about the future. These friends or family members are important, and they should be involved in each step of the process and have their needs addressed earlier rather than later as they are the cornerstone of good dementia care management.

Moving forward

With technological advances people with a dementing illness are being diagnosed much earlier. The model of care that has been most frequently adopted in the past has been that of a person with a physical disability or major physical debilitating illness that requires someone else to do things that the person cannot do for themselves. Unfortunately, this model of care has often meant that the carer inadvisably assumes responsibility for the person with a dementing illness too early, and often inappropriately.

Frequently, the needs and wants of the carer also get lost. The sufferer's life is taken over, often out of misguided love or duty. Unexpressed fears, and reactions to the anticipated grief that lies ahead, can also complicate the issue. To be fair, everybody has done it, got on with the 'doing' or being busy, as a way of coping when they feel overwhelmed by new or different situations. People will do what they know.

Carers historically were viewed as people who did not have the illness and therefore were well. This separation of the two people created a gulf, that, until now, has not been adequately bridged.

The contributions of relationships

When any problem occurs in a family all its members are affected in some way. In the past, the medical profession and psychologists have separated patients from their families. Problems were seen as private. In the late 1970s there was a shift in thinking as it was felt that this view ignored the contributions of relationships.[1] The shift was to a systemic view that included all the family. This change in thinking occurred when individuals were seen to be not improving, causing therapists to look for an external influence.

The family system

The family or the couple is a system. Lions, tigers and elephants all group in families and have certain behavioural characterisitics that are part of their lifestyle. Each animal group has its own system or way of doing things. There may be different families of elephants that live in one area, but each family will have its own pecking order depending on the circumstances that occur within that family. However, when smaller groups are studied by scientists they frequently discover that each animal has its own set of behaviours that impacts on others in the herd.

A system is an organised combination or assembly of things for working together. The family or the couple is a complex system. There are many levels of interaction within the system that influence and affect the behaviour of each individual.

The discovery that interpersonal relationships between family members had an important impact upon a person's problems was the origin of family (or systemic) therapy. This recognised the fact that there are many forces between people, as well as within people, that shape the life experiences of each person.

It is well known that within the environment the relationship between plants, animals, agriculture, insecticides and their toxicity to plants, waterways, trees and the ecosystems are all interrelated. All animals and mammals need each other to survive. They do not exist in isolation. People are very similar in that they form groups called families. Each family has its own set of beliefs, values, rules, expectations and behaviours that govern its internal operation. Similarly, each person within the family has their own set of multiple experiences. If only one aspect of the experience is focused upon and other experiences are ignored, the bigger picture is lost.

'When...spread into other fields, like medicine, it no longer seemed reasonable to focus on only one aspect of a problem or illness without taking into account other relevant variables. Just providing treatment of a disease without treating the whole person is no longer considered viable in general medical practice.'[2]

It would be too simplistic to assume that all families who have a person with a dementing illness were perfect or totally happy prior to the diagnosis. The most stable cohesive families will be challenged.

If the underlying issues in the relationship between the carer and the patient can be improved/supported in the early stages, it would greatly improve the quality of life for both parties and for the family.

Two of the core tenets of systems thinking are that one cannot *not* communicate and that all behaviour has a message. The carer can influence the behaviour of the person with dementia, as the person with dementia can influence or trigger the carer's behaviour. Any family structure potentially holds both the capacity to hurt or help a family member. Therefore care, support and equal involvement from the outset is vital. It is not the number of people in the family, or the type or culture of the family, it is how the family functions in terms of communication, adaptability, cohesiveness, problem solving and how people feel about other family members.

Pre-diagnosis behaviour

Subtle changes in a person's behaviour can occur some years prior to diagnosis. The undiagnosed person and their partner, or some other person in the family, frequently reports the experience of trying to make sense at the time of these unexplained changes—ordinary little things that are slightly skewed such as taking a different street home, forgetting an important date, writing lists, forgetting to give phone messages or repeating a message. These actions mainly concern short-term memory. The people are usually aware of the little niggles, or even experience some anxiety or confusion.

Both parties can experience changes to the relationship. Both parties can experience the anger and frustration caused by some or all of the early symptoms of the disease. One, or both, will eventually look for solutions to the changes that are occurring. Distress at some level will be registering, either consciously or unconsciously, for both parties. Alternatively a family member, a workmate or a friend may raise the alarm. These independent observers can see that there are two people who need help and support, collectively not independently. In fact, the more family members are involved, the better, as they all have a role to play in the ensuing outcome.

Medical intervention, when it occurs, is often viewed as the starting point for changes in the family. However the few years prior to the diagnosis also need to be considered, because it is at this time that the partner or family member may experience a kaleidoscope of emotional feelings and stress. These often remain ill-defined, unspoken and unwitnessed in the early part of the journey. The degree of this stress is generally only recognised much later, when the carer is feeling out of control.

Equal involvement

The parties involved when a person has dementia need to have an equal involvement in the early part of the journey in order to provide them with a structure or solid foundation upon which to build. It will also enable them to protect their emotional investments for as long as possible, and resolve any outstanding issues by encouraging a change in perspective for both parties. This allows both parties to maintain a level of interdependence for a much longer period. They can be empowered by information, consultation, resources and support. They can learn to live each day as fruitfully as possible. They can focus on the positive aspects of life, and know that there is a shared understanding both on a personal and professional level.

The notion of equal involvement and equal need for support from the outset changes the dynamics from the 'one up, one down' position. Shifting the focus from the singular to the plural creates a pool of light that identifies at least two people of equal importance at the time of diagnosis, instead of it being a case of the carer living in the shadows until a crisis occurs. This simple recognition of an equal need for care has the major advantage of reducing the level of guilt and disappointment that frequently occurs later, when the family carer reluctantly realises via a depressive episode or physical illness that they cannot cope.

The disadvantages of unequal involvement

For years carers have stayed behind the scenes, as they often believe that there is no cure or treatment options for a dementing illness. Consequently they adopt a well-worn adage of just 'getting on with it', coping the best way that they can. There is a strong tendency for a carer to use the same strategies to care for the person with dementia as they might use to care for a person with a physical illness. In the early stages of the disease this is unwarranted and often unwanted.

It might go unacknowledged that the carer will definitely have needs of their own while they are caring for a person with dementia. Carers may, as a result, slide silently and subtly into some or all of the following roles, depending on the level of support and enthusiasm of other family members. At times the carer will be a homemaker, a taxi service, a financial controller, a logistics manager, a domestic strategist or a soother of unhappy souls, while at other times they might be the solo breadwinner, the guardian angel for the person with the illness, a mouthpiece (when people ask 'How is Jack?', and Jack is standing right alongside) or a medical and pharmaceutical assistant.

If no opportunity is provided for the new carer to be heard or to share the reality of the changes within the relationship or changes with the family, job, income and future plans, where do these thoughts and feelings go? It is most likely that they transfer to anger, tears, frustration and emotional fragility on some days. They may manifest themselves as a depressive episode, which is most unfortunate as depression is a very complex disorder.

When a study compared those giving care to a person with Alzheimer's disease to a non-caregiving person of similar ages it was found that the caregivers of people with cognitive impairment reported angry feelings, including a tendency to shout and throw things.[3]

This is usually the time when a medical file is begun for a carer at the doctor's office as there is now a recognisable, treatable disease: depression. Alternatively, another file should be opened much earlier at the time of diagnosis that notes the social, educational and emotional needs of the carer.

Multiple benefits of equal involvement

The benefits for equal involvement for the *patient* include:

- The patient feels more supported when the carer is confident and is aware of a realistic health care alternative.
- The patient can relax and focus on their own needs without having to worry about, or be involved in, the blurring of the two roles, which at the time of diagnosis are vague.
- The patient knows that the person who provides care will be cared for as well. The family carer is often the most valuable asset that the person with dementia has in terms of continued support.
- Patients often express anxiety regarding the needs of their carer, particularly if they are not in good health. In some circumstances the person diagnosed has to become the main provider of physical care for both parties.
- Strategies that reduce stress are invaluable for the patient in terms of their cognitive function.
- Both the physical and mental health of the family carer is paramount to the wellbeing of the person with the dementing illness, as they require support for the isolation and social stigma that still abides in our society. They need a safe and predictable environment to enable them to optimise their functionality.

- Experiencing the feeling that they will not be abandoned greatly reduces the anxiety they often express in private to the professional involved. The overt acceptance of the relationship by others is reassuring.
- The patient has the opportunity to share aspects of their identity and personal history prior to diagnosis, which adds a meaningful dimension and personal point of reference for conversations.

The benefits of equal involvement for the *family carer* include:

- The family carer, from the point of diagnosis, feels of equal value and gains verification of the importance of the role.
- The family carer has an individual identity distinct from that of the patient.
- The family carer's needs can be freely expressed, instead of being held in only to resurface later.
- The family carer knows that a professional person is available for them, providing legitimacy for their concerns around the time of diagnosis and beyond.
- There is a professional service to answer the many questions that are frequently asked of a family member who may not have the correct answers.
- The family carer knows that there is professional support that can provide an opportunity to express their anticipatory or disenfranchised (unacknowledged by society or often the family) grief.

The benefits of involvement of both the *carer and the patient* with professionals including doctors, pharmacists, occupational therapists, nurses, physiotherapists, community health workers, educators, psychologists, community service managers, and counsellors will:

- Provide a much wider perspective with which to view the situation, instead of the lineal view of cause and effect.
- Establish a point of reference for both the patient's and the carer's care. When referrals occur, both people are referred; that is, the

patient for management, and the carer for support from the early stages.

- Provide information for other professional staff in the community who will be involved later.
- Reduce the need for multiple service providers.
- Provide a reference point for outside referral to other services, such as counselling or education about the condition. Seminars are considered to be important for both parties when the need arises, as they will have an established rapport with the professional person and be more likely to attend a recommended service.
- Promote mental health and engender confidence via the notion of individuality. This can be fostered so both can have appropriate and confidential opportunities to be heard and understood.
- Enable doctors who are aware of a diagnosis of dementia to inform hospital staff at the time of admission. Even if there is a subtle problem, it may affect how the person with dementia responds to anaesthetics and how the person with dementia responds in the course of treating other medical conditions.
- Enable the carer to distinguish themselves from the patient on all levels. Ultimately, survival and mastery of the journey for both parties depends on this ability.

8. The Living with Memory Loss Program

THE LIVING WITH MEMORY LOSS PROGRAM HAS BEEN WIDELY adopted in Australia (the model used here) since 1997. There are plans to adopt similar programs based on this model, in Europe. These programs have been developed specifically for the needs of the newly diagnosed person and a support person. Ideally the support person would be a partner, close relative or a friend who would be involved in the care of the person as the disease progresses. The purpose is to provide people with essential information, support and a safe environment to discuss personal issues and develop friendships with people in a similar situation.

The Living with Memory Loss Program courses are held at the Alzheimer's Association in each capital city and in some rural areas. The average length of the course is between six and eight weeks held on one day per week for two hours. The course is then followed up by an ongoing early stage group for people with a dementing illness and their carers. These groups are either combined or held separately.

The courses have been available for the past three years and originally were modelled on Robyn Yale's work in America, where she runs support groups for people with Alzheimer's disease.[1] In Australia we have incorporated all kinds of dementing illness, not only Alzheimer's disease. We have also provided a diversional therapy component where the person with a dementing illness's strengths are assessed and enhanced.

The following is an excerpt from a letter from a carer following the course.

> *When he was first diagnosed, I sought support from our local Alzheimer's support group. But I also felt that he himself needed support... He has enjoyed sharing with the only people who really understand—fellow sufferers. Just being able to talk to someone else who understands when the words won't come or if you get lost in telling a story. For myself, being in a small constant group has certainly been a big help. Our partners are all similar ages so we have shared, been educated, been comforted... The program is a big step forward in the care of people with early stage dementia.[2]*

The last five years have seen major changes to the information, support and specific programs available to people who have recently been diagnosed with dementia. It is no longer necessary for people to try to cope without support. One of the concerns for people living with dementia is that the people around them will not understand the changes that are happening. This is the crux of the problem. Changes occur in all aspects of a person's life, and the only thing that looks the same is the outward appearance of the person with dementia.

Acceptance of the diagnosis

The first challenge for the support person is not only to admit that there is a diagnosis but to begin to accept the changes, which can be exceedingly difficult. The degree of acceptance directly influences the benefits to be gained from the program by both parties.

Assessing the level of acceptance is important for both the person with dementia and the family because non-acceptance is loaded with communication difficulties. One of the ways in which to gauge the level of acceptance of the dementia is to step back from the behaviour and step forward to the person. Stepping back means that you no longer ask questions such as: 'Why did you do that? Why did you lose the keys? Why did you lose the car? Why did you forget the apples when I gave you a list? Why did you go to the wrong bank again? Why did you double-book yourself? Why aren't you interested in the children or me? Why didn't you check the change? Where did you leave your wallet? Why don't you listen? How could you get lost? You have driven this road a thousand times.' There is no answer to the 'why' question if something is different from the usual. That is what it is—different. Normal points of reference and practices in everyday living will change, so when family members try to keep things the same then frustration levels will rise. As one person with dementia explained:

> When I am out and about or I am with other people I don't have to think about having dementia, as they do not focus on it like my wife does. For a while I can feel normal. When I am with her she will say, 'But you must remember…this or that or so and so.' I get so angry I could blow my stack when I am told that I must remember something that I obviously do not. When put into this position you have nothing in your arsenal to repudiate the claim. It is a total blank. I just look at her and rage on the inside that she is so stupid to keep on with this. 'You should or must remember this.' She knows I have dementia. Or maybe she *forgets!*

Learning about how to cope with dementia is a new skill, unfortunately it does not come within the general run of life's experience. It could be equated to learning a new computer program but with a lifetime of emotional attachment thrown in. In a recent radio interview, a registered nurse admitted that when her mother was diagnosed with dementia she knew nothing about the disease and went on to describe the difficulties her family experienced because her mother did not admit that she had a problem. This led to many painful situations.

So what can be done when the person will not accept that they have dementia? One way is to learn as much as you can about how and what dementia is. Knowing why some people with a dementing illness will not or cannot acknowledge that they have a problem is part of the learning process for carers and their families.

Families can learn how to work around the denial or lack of insight and reduced judgment that is caused by this unseen brain damage. This can be hard to put into practice when the person still looks the same.

Family members know there is a diagnosis but still need to set up little tests for the person with dementia to check their own reality, because the behaviour changes they observe are often inconsistent. A test can sound something like this: 'But Dad, you must remember, you only told us yesterday. Go and find it—it is in the same place as always. You should try and remember. I am not going to tell you again—you go and have a think about it!' or, 'Mum, this is Susie, she is your granddaughter, you must remember her!' What needs to be learnt is knowing how, why and when to step back, so that perspective can be gained. Imagine if no one was required to take a driving test or learn the rules of the road: there would be chaos.

The basis of the program

The key areas of difference between mainstream support groups and Living with Memory Loss groups is that the latter groups lay the foundation in terms of understanding what dementia is, how it affects the sufferer and how it affects the carer, friend or family. In Living with Memory Loss groups people with dementia and a family member attend a program designed to meet their particular needs. The people with dementia meet in a 'closed' group to discuss their individual needs while the carers meet in another room to discuss their issues. In mainstream support groups only the carers or family members meet.

Support groups invite carers who may be caring for a person anywhere from the early stages through to nursing home placement and afterwards. People come into the group at any point in time or for any length of time. Support groups have long been a life raft for carers. Carers who begin with a Living with Memory Loss program are starting from the beginning and strong bonds are formed as they share similarities each week. Often a story about a particularly stressful event is shared and the group has the ability to see the funny side. For example:

> *Christine went outside to the garden and set John up with a hedge cutter. She went to great lengths to explain that he was safe as there were circuit breakers on the electrical cords so he could just do what he wanted to. She exited, as she did not want to look as if she was his supervisor. A while later she was called because the machine was not working. Upon examination she discovered that he had cut through the electric cord, and her much loved hedge that had been nurtured for years had been redesigned. 'It looked like a bloody pineapple and he looked so bewildered!'*

The group cracked up with laughter. The sense of connectedness with members and having your experience validated is part of the power of group participation. Not only was Christine sharing her experience, she was demonstrating a valuable lesson about the need to be creative in one's approach to care.

The program

This section examines the impact of dementia on the person and how the program will operate for them.

The following is a guide only as to what you may expect from attending a Living with Memory Loss Program.

- To be accepted for who you are, a unique and valuable individual.
- To acquire information that you can use in your daily life.
- To be heard and supported appropriately.
- To have privacy to share with your group any issues that you consider important.
- To participate in decisions affecting current and future care for people with early stage dementia.
- To offer your life experiences to support other people in similar situations, if you choose.
- To provide family members with the opportunity to learn about dementia and how it affects you and your relationships with them.
- To be connected to people and an ongoing supportive environment.
- To connect with other families, volunteers and staff from the Alzheimer's Association.

The list has been formulated in conjunction with people who have completed the program and provided valuable feedback, irrespective of whether they attended the sessions alone or with a partner. If a support person such as a friend, spouse, child or neighbour is available to attend these groups as well, it is extremely helpful.

Each group will have its own individual characteristics. If further information is requested, trained group leaders will arrange special sessions after the group. The sessions cover the information and the adaptations generally needed to make the required adjustments.

Personhood

People have different personalities before they develop dementia and, because many different illnesses cause dementia, there are many variables that have to be taken into consideration when a specific program is offered to people. The uppermost priority is that people must be treated as individuals, not as a group simply because they each have a diagnosis of dementia. In noting and endorsing very important individual differences, the specific program aims to be flexible, specialised and person centred.

Since there is no one specific illness called dementia, people who attend these groups will have different illnesses as well as a diversity of backgrounds and interests. It is very clear that people in the early stage of Alzheimer's disease still have memory: 'and we need to find ways of enabling people to live with the disease by helping them to focus on their strengths and capacities rather than on their losses and on their illness'.[3]

Dr Tom Kitwood, a world-famous dementia expert, along with others developed the idea of 'personhood'. This means that as well as the medical contributions, there needs to be a fundamental shift in thinking:

> Instead of seeing a set of deficits and damages awaiting systematic assessment and careful management, which effectively turns the person into an object, we need to see the person as a whole. This does not deny that there is a dementing illness but sets it in a social context rather than a medical one. One understands the person's dementia as the result of complex interactions between their physical health, their biography or life history, their social psychology (the network of their social relationships) and their neurological impairment.[4]

All these factors make a person who they are. To concentrate on just one factor, without proper regard for the others, is to treat the sufferer as less than a whole person. This concept allows a breath of fresh air in, to provide a sense of hope and difference to the previously held model of negativity and foreboding. Furthermore, if you take the view that everyone is going to die sooner or later, and it is only a matter of time before diagnosis, it makes much more sense to live one day at a time in the most positive way. Pessimism robs all of us of the here and now experience.

Origins

Specific programs for people with early stage dementia began in Australia late in 1997. In the Australian Capital Territory (ACT), Christine Bryden approached the then President of the ACT Alzheimer's Association with an offer of facilitating a support group for people diagnosed with dementia to be conducted under the auspices of the association.

Bryden had been diagnosed with early stage dementia and she had the fortitude to attempt to create change for herself and for others. She was a young scientist who, when diagnosed, found no help forthcoming as she did not fit into the known criteria for people with dementia. Following her diagnosis, Christine said:

> *I did try ringing the Alzheimer's Association, I tried going into it, and they said, 'Is it your father or mother or...' and I said 'Don't worry,' and put down the phone. I did not phone again for another three years, because the expectation was that I would not ring, I would be incapable one day. I had just had the diagnosis the previous day. I was a single parent with four children at that time and was desperate for support and information.*

Christine's approach to the association was timely, as it coincided with their idea to set up services both for people with dementia and for their carers. Christine's group in Canberra has been designed on a needs basis for people with dementia; it differs from other groups in that it is designed for the person with dementia and is open ended, lasting longer than the normal six to eight week programs.

Bryden has continued to do groundbreaking work in the field of dementia in Australia. She writes sensitively and compassionately about her journey in her book *Who Will I Be When I Die?*. At an interview conducted in March 2000, Christine said:

> *The person with dementia is cognitively impaired—what does that mean? Are they cognitively impaired and their brain is scrambled*

so that we can't relate to them, or are they cognitively impaired because we can't relate to them because they can't communicate with us. What is the real barrier? I see myself stumble for words and I see my friends stumble for words. I realise that they know what they want to say but they can't say it. Therefore, in my view, we are not cognitively impaired, but communication impaired.

Communication impairment is the essence of poor relationships. In many cases, people with dementia are left out, stigmatised and devalued because society, friends and families do not understand the challenges faced hourly as they attempt to communicate.

I say to husbands and wives of people with dementia that some-how they underestimate the effort that their partner is making just to get through every day. What if they had a missing leg? You would be really proud of them, you know. They might stuff up, but gee, they have got through the day. If I had an obvious dis-ease certainly people would be far more appreciative of how I was coping…but you can't walk around waving your CAT scan.

How to join a Living with Memory Loss group

It is usually a potential family carer who will seek information for the person with memory problems. In the first instance you can obtain information about the groups via the Alzheimer's help line in your nearest capital city. You may then choose to call the contact person for more information. The sufferer needs to have had a diagnosis of dementia and acknowledge that they have a memory problem and be willing to find helpful ways to live with it. It will not always be as clear-cut as this, where the person can talk about their problems or about the illness. When a person adamantly denies that they have a problem, it is inappropriate to coerce them into being part of a group that they clearly do not want to be part of. Generally, both the carer and the person with dementia will be invited for an interview.

Criteria for memory loss group participants

They must:

- have been assessed or diagnosed as having Alzheimer's disease or one of the related dementias;
- acknowledge the changes to memory;
- understand the implications of the diagnosis;
- be able to talk about what this means to them;
- be able to express their feelings about it;
- want to join the group.[5]

The interview

The first part of the interview usually involves meeting with the group facilitator to have the goals and purpose of the group explained and to answer any questions.

In the second part of the interview the person with dementia and the family member will be interviewed separately, to clarify independently the expectations and insights that they have about the disease and what they hope to achieve by attending the group. It is important for everyone to know that this is not a test, and there are no right answers; it is more about getting to know each other, which is helpful if there are private issues that require individual attention. A time will be made outside the group sessions to address those personal issues that people may not feel comfortable addressing in a group. For instance:

- An ill parent who requires the assistance of a support person, and who also wants to support the person with dementia.
- Adult children having marital or relationship issues with which they are not coping.
- Adolescent children having difficulties accepting the diagnosis.
- Relatives living overseas.
- Financial problems brought about through unplanned retirement or loss of a job.

- Pre-existing marital or relationship issues.
- Conflict within the family.
- Family member denying that there is a diagnosis.
- A parent or in-law has been taken into the family home and there is ambivalence about the arrangement with one or more family members.

The third part of the interview is the completion of some basic forms that give demographic data and identify any special medication that either party is taking and any support services involved.

People with mild cognitive impairment have been found to gain the most benefit from the group. One standardised tool used to measure mild cognitive impairment is the Folstein Mini Mental State Examination (MMSE see Appendix III).

Usually the MMSE is conducted along with other tests as part of the diagnostic procedure and, if possible, a copy should be brought with you to the interview. Alternatively the person who has done the testing can be contacted for the results. If the results are unavailable the MMSE will be done at the interview. MMSE is used to gain a benchmark, as the model currently in use for the Living with Memory Loss Program requires a score of 18 or above out of 30.

Group members are asked to be involved in an evaluation program, which provides important feedback to participants and the group facilitators so they can adjust the program if needed in the future.

Information regarding the time, place and date that the program will commence will be given. There are usually around six to eight couples per program.

The agenda

The series begin with a meeting of group facilitators and participants to give an overview of the day's session and give notice of any official business, then the groups go to their separate areas for about one and a half hours. The groups then reconvene for coffee and socialisation.

The sessions usually last about two hours each week over six to eight weeks.

Each area may have a slightly different group format; however, the essential areas that will be covered are as follows.

Living with Memory Loss Program for people with dementia

Session one: What is dementia?

Following group introductions and housekeeping matters the group discusses its understanding of what dementia is. The focus is on a general overview of dementia, which includes understanding that it is the result of brain damage caused by many diseases, the most common being Alzheimer's disease, or multiple strokes. Participants share information about occupations, past and present interests, and which aspects of these they have retained. The focus is on healthy coping skills that can be encouraged and expanded. Dementia is caused by deterioration of parts of the brain. It is not a failure of the person.

Session two: Diagnosis and beyond— what is it like to live with dementia?

This session will cover things such as a participant's experience regarding the process of obtaining the diagnosis; life issues that occurred along the way; changes that have occurred; the differences in progress and symptoms; the impact of the disease on themselves; coping with memory loss, concentration and difficulty thinking some things through; and the loss of interest in things previously enjoyed and difficulties in performing some tasks.

In this session, helpful practical strategies for dealing with the difficult changes that dementia brings will be provided as well as contributions received from the group members—who are the experts.

- Write reminders in diaries or calendars.
- Keep a white board on the refrigerator with the day's date and appointments written clearly in point form.
- Try to keep things such as car keys, glasses, wallet or handbag, pencils or pens or the telephone index in set places.
- Keep a writing pad beside the phone.
- Keep to known routines for activities such as breakfast, showering, the daily walk.
- Set days for appointments if possible, and ask others to remind you as near as possible to the event.
- Talk to yourself—it helps to get information in.
- Have photographs of the family on the refrigerator, with their names written below. This is important for new family members and grandchildren.
- Have clocks positioned near the telephone, refrigerator and your favourite chair.
- Ask for the alarm clock to be set for a certain time with a note attached telling you what you need to remember at that time.

To cope with changes in concentration:

- Break information down into small steps.
- Deal with the small bits, and then think about it a step at a time.
- Turn off distractions like the TV or radio.
- Ask people to repeat information clearly.
- Write things down.
- Avoid loud shopping malls at the busy times of the day.
- Take your time and avoid being hassled.
- If reading becomes a problem, try talking books.

If you are having difficulties with familiar tasks:

- Break the task down into small steps.
- Write down the steps or ask someone to type them out for you.
- Ask someone to prompt you about what step comes next.

- Remind people not to take over the tasks; you just need a little support.

The session ends on a positive note as participants share personal strategies on ways that they have learnt to overcome their short-term memory problems.

Session three: Focusing on the positive

This session is most often a combined group of both sufferers and carers. A medical practitioner is invited to give an overview of the more common forms of dementia and to answer any questions. If time permits, the groups will reconvene in their respective areas to discuss the outcome of the medical session.

If time permits, this session also looks at people's likes. What do they enjoy? In the past, who has helped with this? How have they done it? Local councils usually have a hive of community activities going on, so how do you access these? People's interests change over time, so having a problem with memory does not mean that there are no activities for you—you can take up painting, walking, swimming classes, Scrabble or historical meandering in your local area. These activities can be done with the support of other people or a family member.

Session four: Relationship changes with family and friends

Every day you use some method of communication to make yourself heard and understood by others. The word 'communication' means to share or exchange common ideas and feelings. This is the opposite of keeping thoughts and feelings to yourself.

Changes to the way you communicate impacts on your relationships and how you feel about yourself. The closer to and safer you feel with the people around you, the more relaxed you can be about adapting to these changes. In Session four some of these changes are reviewed and solutions sought for carers and families. Areas to explore include:

- Do you have to rely on other people more now than in the past?
- What has that been like?
- Since your diagnosis, do people treat you the same or differently at home, at church, in your local community or in your street?
- What has been the most difficult aspect of having memory problems in terms of communication with your family or friends?
- What are some of the most helpful things that your partner does for you?
- What are some of the difficult things that your partner does?
- What would you like to change or improve about the way in which your partner communicates with you?
- What has it been like giving up some of your previous roles in the family, for example, managing the financial affairs?

When a person's communication is impaired and their needs are not heeded and go unexpressed, the result may often be some form of negative behaviour. The most prevalent negative emotions are anger or depression. The event that caused the distress may be forgotten, but the associated feelings remain. Reduced or poor communication can result in not being asked; not being involved in decision making; being ignored or not heard; being spoken about as though you were invisible; feeling that your life is being taken over; people minimising what you are going through; being patronised; or struggling between trying to stay as functional as possible and needing to accept help in some areas.

The following strategies to improve communication were suggested by people with dementia who attended these groups.

- Don't let us feel like a failure.
- Remind us that we are very much part of the past, the present and the future.
- Consider our memory problems and speak simply and clearly.
- Reduce distractions like the noise of the TV and radio.
- Record information in our diary for us.

- Keep notices around the house up to date.
- Remind us to use our diary and read notices on the calendar or whiteboard.
- Allow us plenty of time for what you have said to be understood. Give us time to sort through words to find the best one.
- Use orientation landmarks such as names and places or events in your opening comments: 'I hear that you are off to Lismore to attend your son Bob's wedding next week' rather than 'When will you be going to your son's wedding?'
- Try to keep us as involved as possible.
- A warm smile and gentle touch on the arm or hand will most often get our attention and it feels good as well.
- We may not have intellectual equity with others to the same level as before, but we still need to have the same right to be treated with dignity.
- We all need human companionship, and that means being involved with daily activities.[6]

Aspects of giving back dignity are discussed here:

> [T]he best assistance is that which is unobtrusive. Helpers who quietly get things done, rather than announcing their efforts, leave a dependent person's pride intact. The indebtedness position is not emphasized, and the carer makes no mention of special accommodations. The fact of helplessness then recedes into the background, where it can reside without harming the person's self esteem.[7]

Session five: Planning for the future

A professional financial adviser is often invited to this session to discuss legal issues for people with dementia and their carers. It is often a combined group.

Some people are great planners, while others have a more laissez-faire approach. One of the major advantages of planning is that you have a say in how, when and where your private affairs will be attended to. Some of these matters will require your immediate attention; others will need careful consideration and discussion before you make a decision.

Finances

Michael Longhurst's publication *The Beginner's Guide to Retirement*[8] and Peter Cerexhe's book *Before and After Retirement*[9] are excellent resources for people making financial decisions around the time of retirement and beyond. If you are in the throes of exiting from the workforce, decisions need to be made about superannuation and financial planning. Choosing a trustworthy financial planner can be a wise investment at this juncture, or you could consult with a financial planner to find out about your entitlements across the full range of government benefits and assistance that are on offer. People who are already retired can access up-to-date information through their local Alzheimer's Association, as the laws are changing continually.

Enduring power of attorney

A power of attorney document gives a person you choose authorisation to act on your behalf to manage your financial affairs. This document is invalid if the sufferer becomes mentally incapacitated. An enduring power of attorney document is the means by which a person can appoint someone whom they trust to act for them should they become mentally incapacitated and unable to look after things themselves at some future time. This could be due to physical problems, loss of mental capacity or something unforeseen such as an accident. It is only possible to grant enduring power of attorney if the person is capable of understanding what it is and what it is intended to do. One excellent website provides a question and answer section that would be useful to read before you go to your solicitor. It will enable you to think things through in your own time and compile a list of your own questions.[10]

Wills

A will is a legal document naming the people you have chosen to receive your assets when you die. Making a will is the only way you can ensure that your assets are distributed according to your wishes.[11] Often people discuss the differences in the costs of making a will; Peter Cerexhe's reply to the question 'Which one will cost me the most?' is 'The one that makes a mistake!' Therefore have your will completed by a professional to ensure your wishes are explicitly written.

Enduring guardianship

The focus of enduring guardianship is on personal or lifestyle care rather than on financial matters. Everybody would like to decide for themselves where they live, who they choose to see, which doctor they go to and what medical treatment they receive. Unfortunately, this is not always possible. Contact your own solicitor or the Alzheimer's helpline on legal and financial matters.

Accommodation

There are now so many housing options for people who no longer have families living at home; some people move into retirement accommodation to avoid the hassle later, while others prefer to live in the same home and have modifications done when required. This is a very personal matter that does warrant discussion with the family, but you should be prudent. If your pets are part of you, then you may choose to stay put. Your neighbourhood and familiarity with your community can be a great source of comfort when you are having problems with your memory. Landmarks in your street or shopping centre can be great aids to your orientation.

Session six: Looking after you

If you don't use it you'll lose it as the old adage says. Staying fit and healthy is all part of looking after yourself. Some activities that you did previously may still be done but you may need some support, for example, playing tennis, bowls or golf and relying on another person to do the scoring.

Some people desire to do an activity but the initiation button in the brain does not fire as well as it did, so this is where they will need some help to get going. Planning and initiation are features that may be reduced in the early stages of dementia, but an informed carer will be able to help you to maintain some of the things that have given you pleasure in the past for a long time to come.

Some people believe that stimulating the brain by learning lists of things and doing memory exercises, games and puzzles will improve brain function. There is no empirical evidence to suggest that these activities improve or slow the progression of the disease after the brain is impaired due to Alzheimer's disease,[12] so I would recommend that people continue to do what they enjoy. Keeping a list of activities in a prominent place in the home can remind both you and other members of the family that there are many choices to be made. Having a family member, a friend or neighbour do some of these activities with you can enhance the pleasure and sense of companionship.

The following is a small list of activities that you may consider doing.

- Reading the newspaper, magazines or books.
- Crosswords, Scrabble, Trivial Pursuit, cards.
- Walking, swimming, dancing, tenpin bowling, lawn bowls.
- Gardening—growing flowers in planter boxes, herb gardens.
- Walking the dog, grooming the dog.
- Painting for pleasure.
- Cooking and sewing.
- Listening to music, going to films.

- Joining a local walking group.
- Doing gentle and continuous exercise with a group or with the aid of a video at home.
- Having a massage just for the pleasure.
- Watching your favourite show on television.
- Attending your local church and being involved in some of the community activities.

Driving

For many people the driver's licence[13] is an important symbol of perceived fitness as a member of the community.[14] While there has been much research on driving and dementia to date, there are no clear guidelines that can be globally applied. The tough question is balancing the issues of risk versus autonomy.

Many older people self-regulate their driving practices in response to their needs and changing abilities. When a person has dementia, self-regulation may only happen spasmodically. Many good and impartial doctors recommend that people with dementia attend a driving test conducted by an occupational therapist; the advantages being that this will provide an objective assessment. Furthermore, an independent person with the appropriate training can do a thorough assessment of the person with dementia without prior judgment. Having a licence revoked by the Road Traffic Authority without prior warning is not helpful. It is better to have made your own decision to be assessed.

Getting a comprehensive assessment in the early stages of dementia will allow the sufferer to understand that, later on, they may have to hand in their licence. Meanwhile, they can feel safe knowing that they have been assessed and their driving skills are acceptable. The occupational therapist will provide support and counselling to people who are assessed as being no longer capable of driving safely. Proposals for alternative strategies for transportation can then be discussed.

Laughter

Laughter is a great leveller. When things happen you have two choices: to laugh or to cry, but we know which one feels the best. Both release endorphins in the brain, which is mentally relaxing. Keeping a sense of humour can be typified by a little story found in a recent issue of the *Apnea News* magazine.[15]

> ### Sad News
>
> I don't usually pass on news like this, but sometimes we need to pause and remember what life is about…
>
> There was a great loss recently in the entertainment world. Larry La Pries, the Detroit native who wrote the song 'Hokey Pokey', died last week at age 83. It was especially difficult for the family to get him in the casket. They put his left leg in and well, things just started to go downhill from there.

At the end of Session six many people make arrangements to meet fortnightly or monthly as a social group. Alternatively, they may form a group requiring additional information on certain topics. Each group becomes independent. Some have coffee mornings and some meet with partners. Some groups of people with dementia meet on a regular basis, as they feel that this is a place of comfort and acceptance where wonderful friendships are made and sustained. The Alzheimer's associations frequently host these meetings as a follow-up program.

Living with Memory Loss Program for carers and support people

One of the reasons that carers go to a different group from the people with dementia is that they have very different needs. Imagine two small lush tropical desert islands near the Great Barrier Reef connected to each other by a sand bar. Both are exposed to the same environmental elements, but what happens on each island is different. The first island may once have had people living on it who had planted certain trees and vegetation because there was fresh water. The second island only has palm trees and inedible tropical vegetation. The sand bar between the two islands represents shared experiences and a sense of connection between each other, but the islands have an identity all of their own.

Carers often hold on to what they know and love about the person with dementia and at the same time are trying to adapt to the often unwanted changes that are occurring without their consent or choice. Life as they had known it has changed. Just how to live with and adjust to these lifestyle changes is what this course is about. Having the benefit of being with people who are in a similar situation provides a sense of connection. It moves from the private and personal to the social and universal sharing of similarities. One of the first challenges for carers is to remain within a family and a relationship that is changing while endeavouring to remain the same person. The aim of this course is about how to bridge this personal and social gap and live with a different perspective and level of understanding of the person with dementia and oneself.

Session one: Introductions and personal overview

Group members are welcomed, and the group rules are established. Basic group rules need to include the following:

- Confidentiality is paramount.
- Each person is entitled to their opinion.
- Each member can use this forum to say anything without fear of criticism or rejection.
- Each person will get a chance to speak.
- This is a safe place for people to share as much or as little as they choose.
- The more that is shared the richer the experience.

This session will centre on personal experiences of the group members. Discussions include 'Am I alone?', 'Am I different?', 'Why are

we here?', 'I don't have the problem, my partner has the problem' and
'What would I like to get out of this group?'.

If time permits the session moves on to:

- Dementia and its history in your life.
- How did the diagnosis occur?
- When did it occur?
- How did you find out about it?
- What did your family do or say about the diagnosis?
- How has your life changed. For example, have you moved house, taken up full-time or part-time work?
- In what way has it affected your life?
- What would you like to take away from this six-week course?

Not all of these questions will be answered in this session and participants will be offered a take-home sheet to complete this personal history session. Some people prefer to reflect upon these issues and return with it the following week. The purpose of this exercise is to provide the opportunity to focus on personal needs. For some people there are many surprises in this first session, the first being to think about what has happened to themselves during the time before and following the diagnosis. Consider these observations:

> *I had never really thought about myself when David was diagnosed. There was so much happening at the time. I remember having a lot of tears and feeling angry, but I could not do that in front of him—he was having enough of his own difficulties.*

> *I kick myself because I should have seen it coming. I feel so stupid. When I remember the arguments that we started to have about money, and the family, and his work. Oh dear!*

> *I cannot come to terms with the fact that I saw my mother cope with this with her mother and now I have to do it. I mean, don't*

get me wrong. I will do it because I love her, but I do remember that my grandmother's behaviour really tried my mother's patience to an unbelievable level.

The ATM machine was really the first thing that I noticed. He said it was broken. At first I just said, 'Typical, these things are good while and when they work.' But after the third time I thought, what is going on here?

I am okay myself, but it is the other people in the family that I am having difficulty with. They just don't want to know. He is their brother and he was always the one that they turned to and now it is his turn and where are they? You would think that he had a contagious disease.

My husband is a wonderful man, but he is having difficulty understanding how I feel about my mum, who has dementia. He doesn't say it in so many words but he will say 'what about our kids, and us?'. I don't know how to manage it all. She needs me now, the kids need me, he needs me. I have to work part-time, and there are just not enough hours in the day.

She is my best friend and I will do or learn anything that I can about how to help her. I want to make every day count for something.

Session two: Expanding knowledge about dementia

In Session two the aspects of the most common diseases that cause dementia and the relationship between the affected parts of the brain and the person's behaviour are discussed. Also covered are facts and figures about dementia worldwide; common myths about dementia; the relationship changes between yourself and your partner/friend/ relative due to the dementia; and common issues such as changes to communication, speech, writing and reading, remembering appointments, apparent lack of initiative, moods swings, distractability, inappropriate behaviours at times and the inability to complete some tasks.

Many myths have evolved over time about dementia. These are singularly unhelpful and need to be addressed. Often, what we believe forms the basis of our behaviour and that of others. Some common myths include:

- Dementia is contagious.
- It only happens to people who have not used their brain.
- It is more likely to occur in developed countries.
- Everyone gets memory problems as they get older.
- Nothing can be done for the person with dementia.
- Relatives of people with dementia are likely to inherit the disease.

Sometimes people are not aware that they even hold beliefs about dementia, so this session is important for helping to separate fact from fiction. It is very empowering for participants, because they can actually see a video with a geriatrician explaining just how the diseased parts of the brain directly affect a person's behaviour. This new knowledge begins to make some sense of the relationship changes that have been occurring and that have frequently caused much distress in families. It clarifies the issue about whether the person with dementia has a choice about using selective memory on occasions. Here you begin to understand how repeating things, raising your voice or expressing your frustration is a futile exercise. Here you can learn to do things differently.

Session three: The medical side of dementia

This may be a combined group or it may be held separately. A medical practitioner gives a brief overview of dementia, including a synopsis of the different causes of dementia. This provides an opportunity for group participants to ask questions about behaviours, anti-dementia drugs, anti-depressant drugs, any other illness that they or the person with dementia has as well as dementia.

It is best to prepare a list of questions for this session, if possible, as most people report that they learned some new information because of the questions that other people asked.

Session four: Looking after yourself

This session links back to Session one, where each person's individual issues can be dealt with more fully. What is happening in your life now is compared with life prior to the diagnosis. What happens on a routine day? What do you do for yourself each week, each day? What comforts you? Partial and total losses are explored, and time, finances, shared hobbies, intimacy, role reversals, friendships new and lost, divided loyalties, work, and fears about the future are discussed.

Each person reviews what is happening to them now, and ways that they can maintain a balance physically, emotionally, psychologically and spiritually are looked at. Each person has the opportunity to share their expertise about time management, self-care, challenges surmounted, strengths, and solutions to some relationship issues.

At this stage people often discuss emotional issues that worry them, for instance anger. The triggers that spark off anger, how it is expressed and what effect it is having are explored and discussed. Instead of being seen as a totally negative experience, anger can alternatively be seen as a 'gift' as it flags a distress signal and highlights the need for support and time out.

Carer burden is a subjective experience. What distresses one person will not affect someone else in the same way. However, lack of time for ourselves can quickly lead to either depression or inappropriate anger which, if ignored, causes untold distress for the carer and most certainly for the person with dementia.

Session five: Planning for the future

This may be a combined group or it may be separate. The topics explained cover finances, power of attorney, wills, accommodation and legal issues as described in Session five of the Living with Memory Loss program for people with dementia (pages 105–107).

Having a combined group has, in general, been a positive experience for couples, as some topics that have been an issue have been better accepted by the person with dementia when raised by a third party. This session is very much focused on the early stages of dementia as this is the time that the person with memory loss can make informed choices about their future. If participants wish to attend another session at a later time, it can be arranged.

Planning for the future involves the following points. Advice can also be sought individually from financial planners and from the Alzheimer's helpline.

- Accommodation, investing, retirement, redundancy and aged care.
- Investment products and how they work, their advantages and disadvantages and the taxation implications.
- The options for carers to work part-time.
- Will the carer be able to return to work?
- Do you have sufficient income and assets to support yourself while providing care?
- If not, will you be eligible for income support from the state or other assistance?
- A fact to consider: only one in every twelve people make plans for their retirement.
- To fund your current lifestyle in your retirement, ideally you would need a lump sum of approximately ten times your current annual salary.
- Why plan? Over 700 000 people in the UK alone have dementia. Dementia affects one in twenty people over the age of sixty-five, and one in five people over the age of eighty.
- A financial strategy is to look at yourself: Where are you now? What are you worth?
- Where are you going? What do you need? What do you want?

The Alzheimer's Association's financial and legal arrangements fact-sheet covers how to arrange the financial and legal affairs of the person with dementia. It will inform you that specific personal issues about wills and family trusts will require a solicitor. The earlier enduring power of attorney, enduring guardianship, wills and living wills are implemented, the better it is, generally, for those involved. The person with dementia must have testamentary capacity for the documents to be deemed legal. Wills have been contested when a will has been changed some years following the diagnosis of dementia; for example, when a parent has remarried and willed the family estate to the new partner.

Session six: Sexuality and intimacy

Participants in this group are generally between forty and eighty years of age.

The intimacy and sexual experiences of older members would generally have been formulated over many years and has either been sustained, maintained or relinquished by life experiences. For example, Bob and Honor have been married for fifty years. Their 'intimacy' (close and warm friendship) may only have been recorded by some tiny sepia photographs in a tired old heavy black paper album that lies gathering dust. The photographs were taken by the professional photographer in town, somewhere outside a significant architectural edifice, where they wore their best clothes for a visit to the city.

This generation grew up with the same sexual make-up as today's wonderful youth but was constrained by a multitude of social mores: the church, family, school and community. Myths were often based on ignorance and shame. There were secret adoptions, and loves lost during the war. There was no abortion on demand, and no reliable contraception. Intimacy and personal wisdom were tightly intertwined.

Life does move on and older people tend to become involved with their family and the community. However, all losses are felt.

When physical or mental changes occur and people are not as actively occupied as before, this can be a time when people revisit those losses. Their reactions are commonly labelled as depression. Furthermore, the cause of the depression is often attributed to living alone, to changes in physical or mental health or because of the inability to form meaningful relationships which are often only a part of deeper issues.

The loss of intimacy as it had previously been known and a change in sexuality is certainly different for this age group than it is for younger members. Acknowledgement and validation of that loss is very therapeutic in helping to resolve the grief and move on to another stage of life.

There are many aspects of a carer's life that require reorganisation. Loss or potential loss of the sexual side of the relationship is a very pivotal event and a significant physical and emotional loss. If left unexpressed it can lead to emotional trauma and depression. It is often thought by family and the medical profession that being a carer in general is the cause of the depression rather than the private and personal issues that are going unaddressed. Loss of sexuality is often laughed about, and no bigger amusement was to be found than in the jokes that circulated when the drug Viagra was launched a few years ago. However, there is a darker side to the loss of libido that is not discussed, acknowledged or mourned appropriately.

Many people's sexual prowess is closely linked with their identity and mental health, so loss of libido can have an inestimable effect on the person with dementia and requires great sensitivity and understanding on the part of the carer. Carers may also suffer the loss of sexual functionality. Some carers have difficulty with the idea of making love to a person who has changed so much, principally because when it is over they may have forgotten. Carers often describe the feeling of being prematurely deserted:

I know that this is ridiculous at my age [seventy-four] but we have always enjoyed a warm and mutually satisfying sexual relationship. It has helped tremendously through some of the difficult times when all we had was each other. He can no longer even hold me, or touch me with any significant meaning. I think it is the loss of exclusivity that I am upset about. He does not treat me any differently to anyone else. I know it is irrational, but it still hurts.

This issue may not affect everybody. Some people have redesigned their lives to include outside interests to take up their time, attention and affection. They redirect their energy and happily reconcile these losses.

Another group that can be affected is those in second or third marriages in later life. This poem, about the cards people are dealt in life expresses one woman's feelings after discovering that her husband had Alzheimer's disease after they had been married for six years.[16]

The prayer of the frog
In the game of cards called life
one plays the hand one is dealt to the best of one's ability.
Those who insist on playing, not the hand they were given but
    the one they insist they should have been dealt—these are
    life's failures.
We were not asked if we would play.
That is not an option. Play we must.
The option is how.[17]

It is not uncommon for newly wed people to find that their partner has early onset or early stage dementia, especially if they are over the age of sixty-five. Sexuality and intimacy is both a very personal issue and a very normal aspect of life. Changes in either affect people's lives significantly. If you realise that there will be changes in libido as part of ageing, you may not be at all worried. Most people have some thoughts about when or how active sexual relationships begin to decline, and if their beliefs and their reality are incongruent then that can become an issue of concern.

The meaning of intimacy for many people is often confused with sexuality in all of its many forms. This can be a cause of much distress, if the carer has experienced a sudden cessation of a previously satisfying sexual relationship. Often what people miss the most is not the act of sexual intercourse but the touching, the holding and the affection that exists between two people. Sometimes a formerly affectionate person will no longer accept affection when they have brain damage.[18]

There is no easy solution to intimacy problems, but you could go and see your partner's doctor and try to find out the exact nature and extent of the brain damage and how it is linked to this part of their changed behaviour. Requesting a one-on-one session with a dementia-specific counsellor to discuss these issues has also proved very helpful for many people.

Ongoing groups

Following the conclusion of these sessions, carer groups often meet on a regular basis to share both personal, social and recreational activities. Forming friendships with people in a similar situation is a new dimension of the support group service.

Some people have never had the opportunity of receiving specific educational, psychosocial support and individual or couple counselling at the beginning of their journey. By the time they sought assistance with their problem they were often isolated and exhausted. When one's emotional resources are low and the needs of care increase, there is little time for seeking out supportive friendships, which can be sustaining for the period and lifelong as a personal investment.

Feedback from discussion groups

Individual feedback from participants is very positive, the highlights being: sharing with others in the same situation, education and support of the facilitators. A summary of participant feedback is included below.

What carers liked most

- Meeting, talking to and the support of the facilitators.
- Sharing with others in the same situation and discussing ways of handling difficult situations.
- Access to medical and legal information.
- The fellowship and friendship of all involved, including staff.
- The consistency of the group.
- The benefit of their partner having contact with other people with dementia.
- Knowledge, education and acceptance.

What people living with dementia liked most

- The casual, relaxed way in which facilitators spoke of the disease and group unity.
- The suggestions for handling difficult times.
- Meeting other people in the same stage of dementia and sharing problems and a laugh.
- Talks by a doctor.
- Opportunities to discuss various topics at their own pace and flexibility to return to previous points.

The components participants found most helpful

- Ongoing support with knowledgeable counsellors.
- Resources—videos, books, other people's experiences with the disease.

- Help sheets and handouts ('a great reference for future needs').
- Library services.
- Legal information.
- 'Every day had something worthwhile to offer.'

Feedback from the diversional therapy component

After completion of the discussion groups, there is a short break followed by an eight to ten week leisure activity program with the diversional therapist for the memory loss group people. The therapist interviews participants prior to the group. The purpose and aim of the group is to explore leisure activities that aim to increase their social network, their confidence and their quality of life.

While the memory loss people attend their group, the carers continue to meet as a self-directed group. If they have any requests for topics to be presented, the facilitator arranges this for them. People attend individual counselling sessions to address particular needs that they feel are not always appropriate for a larger group.

All of the groups elected to have monthly reunions to maintain the support network and facilitate ongoing education about all the services offered by the Alzheimer's Association.

Each service that sets up a Living with Memory Loss program will have issues such as appropriate venues, available staff, length of course and timing of follow-up sessions before people are reassessed. This is an evolving process and what I have outlined here is only a guide. As new information and treatments become available, changes will take place in the content, duration and follow-up of the program. What will not change is the need to involve families from the point of diagnosis, the need for equal partnerships and the support required to adapt to the changes.

part three

The psychology of caring

9 The family

FAMILIES ARE THE STRUCTURE UPON WHICH GOOD CARE IS BUILT FOR the person with dementia. Each person in the family will have a different view of care: some will offer hands-on care, others technical or emotional support and others will do nothing. Often it is the most unlikely person in the family that will take on the greatest level of care, or be extremely supportive to the primary carer. Irrespective of the role adopted, each person will be affected in some way. Often this depends on the relationship they have with the person with dementia.

Changes in roles and relationships

At sometime or other everyone mentions the word 'family'. In that word alone there are many variables, but for convenience of communication the word is used as if its meaning is understood. The old myth about all families being a tight-knit, cohesive unit that will defend the rights of other members to the death seems a far cry from the compilations of people who see themselves today as families.

The term 'nuclear family' was coined in the 1970s to depict families that were a primary social unit, one with two parents and their offspring, functioning as a single entity. The extended family included the nuclear family with blood relatives, sometimes spanning three generations.[1] This is the family often quoted as the cornerstone of support for a person with a dementing illness. Where do the single-parent households, the same-sex partners, the unmarried people and the people who live alone fit today in the assumed notion of family?

To simplify matters the definition of family is taken as meaning 'A basic unit of society, characterised as one whose members are economically and emotionally dependent on one another and are responsible for each other's development...currently, in our society the traditional definition of the family is undergoing many changes because of the emerging prominence of alternative lifestyle.'[2] This is not a perfect definition of a family but the aim is to include all people, both biologically and socially connected to the person with dementia and who, behaviourally, operationally and spiritually, view themselves as family.

Role reversal can be one of the greatest changes in a family member's position; it may come about unconsciously or consciously depending on the situation and the beliefs about care and the age of the person for whom care is required. Changes to one's role and identity are by far the most difficult challenges to be met in the early stages of dementia, as they occur over time and are rarely thought about.

Over the years people develop a way of 'being' in their relationships. Families can hold similarities in terms of what is measurable statistically, but the essence of what transpires and how it transpires within the private realms of the family and their relationship is absolutely unique. It is the 'into me, see' or intimacy issues that are often first affected in the early stages of dementia, as both parties are trying to adapt to the changes that are occurring in their lives. Throwing a stone into a pond is one way of conceptualising this. First there is the impact of the stone hitting the water, followed by the ripples which spread in ever-widening circles. The first impact often emerges softly or hesitantly—as do those little things such as a forgotten appointment.

My sister lives in the country and I had phoned her the night before to confirm our appointment at 9.30 am at Central Railway Station. She laughed and said 'I am all packed and ready.' I arrived there at about ten past nine and waited. Trains came and went and I waited and waited. She has always been a real stickler for appointments and being on time. I then checked with the stationmaster just in case the train was late. I began looking on other platforms, in the ladies' toilet and back to the station. I waited for an hour and a half. I began to feel sick. I phoned her home and there was no reply. I phoned the dentist where she had an appointment at 11 o'clock. I was beside myself. I phoned on and off for the rest of the day. Then about 4 pm she finally answered the phone and told me that she had been out for a lovely day with the lady next door. I did not know whether to scream at her or cry. I knew now that we definitely had a big problem.

Changes to the family structure

Any changes to the family structure challenge your own sense of who you are. Families are now faced with the unprecedented challenges of balancing the needs of several generations that do not usually dwell in the same household. Families now also provide the majority of caregiving for people with a dementing illness. To have a relative with a dementing illness can compound the problems that already exist within many families today, causing depression, workplace pressure and family frictions.

When a diagnosis of dementia occurs, the family has to adjust and reshape itself. Each individual member will have a different reaction to the news of a diagnosis. Some family members may not be told of the diagnosis while others, even if told, will choose 'not to know'. Families handle new information very differently depending on the content of the information and what effect it will have on them individually or collectively, and depending on what changes they can or will choose to make. Choosing not to know may be a way of coping with information that is too hurtful, involves too much responsibility, or can be too disruptive to a person's or family's life. A family friend saw 'choosing not to know' as follows.

> *Three of her children were here for dinner last week and they have a very poor idea of just how difficult life is for her. They know that she has been diagnosed, and she has given them joint power of attorney and fixed up her financial affairs. Because she is on her own turf they seem to think that she is fine, which she isn't. I don't want them to think that I am just a Svengali figure. There is a frenetic euphoria when they visit; it is as if they desperately want things to be normal. They have their own families and they don't want to know any bad news.*

This observer felt that the family were colluding, as not one of them appeared to want to be involved or to make changes that could incorporate their mother.

Family members may take up a position that is different to the one previously held. This change in role is influenced by gender, geography, position held in the family, availability, beliefs about care, economic situation, physical health, mental health, caring dispositions, living arrangements and life stage, family alignments and political affiliations within the family. In one blended family the husband, who had been married to his current wife for fifteen years, suffered from dementia. His wife said:

> *When we received the diagnosis, it is as if we realigned with our respective kin looking for solace and support. His family surrounded him, and I went to my only brother. For a time it felt like I was an outsider, despite the fact that we had been married for fifteen years. He turned to his children, and they towards him. I wept silently on the wings of that stage. His children will never know what it felt like to be on the outside.*

Selection of a carer

A primary carer is selected either voluntarily or, in time, will be conscripted into the carer role depending on the selection process adopted by the family. The selection process does not necessarily result from objective family discussion. These quotes were taken from carer interviews on the issue of carer choice and duty.

> *Basically it happened by circumstance. I have always lived at home with Mum and Dad and I did it because the other siblings were not able to. It was not a matter of choice.*

> *I am the only daughter with four brothers and it had always been a 'given' that I would be the carer. The fact that I had three children of my own was neither here nor there.*

> *It just happened, I don't recognise myself as volunteering. I just did it. I suppose if you wanted to volunteer you put your hand up and do it. That was not how it was for me.*

What is really meant by family caregiver?

Caring can be viewed as a specific activity that includes everything you do to maintain, continue and repair your 'world' so that you can live in it as well as possible. That world includes your body, yourself and your environment, all of which you seek to interweave in a complex, life-sustaining web.[3]

This general overview of caring sets the scene to explore further the specifics of caring for a person with dementia. Taking the view that caregiving involves both 'activity' and 'emotions', it would be reasonable to note that the carer's whole being is involved when caregiving for another person. Caregiving involves three major components: responsibility, choice, and the customary expectations in relationships.

Caring has been distinguished as two separate meanings 'caring about' from that of 'caring for'.[4] 'Caring for' tends to have a more practical application, as opposed to 'caring about' which involves the carer's feelings for another person. Parenting is a caregiving task, as it involves both doing and feeling. However, care for a person with dementia is different, as the tasks required go beyond the normal reciprocities between adults.[5]

After the diagnosis of a dementing illness the overall responsibility needs to be allocated to someone. People from outside the family can offer services such as driving or filling out forms, but the overall responsibility for the person's health and wellbeing will be allocated to the primary caregiver to coordinate.

When a person from outside the family volunteers to care, they have a choice about how much care to provide and they have the option of when to withdraw their services. This does not in any way minimise the value of care offered by willing volunteers; rather, it highlights the differences regarding choice.

Choice about caring has important ramifications for families. It is very different to choosing from among the alternatives available to people who volunteer their services. A family member has little choice about the onset of the disease or the length of their caregiving duties. Lack of choice about caregiving in a family can disempower some carers who feel they have to put their lives on hold and forgo activities for an undetermined length of time.

Each family develops comfort zones around personal levels of distance and closeness between individual family members. For example, some families consider it normal behaviour to chat to each other in the bathroom while one is showering. Other families experience difficulties in open displays of affection. Some families phone each other weekly, whereas other families 'expect' some form of contact each month or each day. When a person with dementia requires caregiving that includes personal care, the issues of what is appropriate often frames the deeper issues of how much closeness or distance is tolerable within the relationship.

Transgression of comfort zones and expectations associated with caregiving often depends on the individual situation. An older couple may have decided that they would reciprocate care for each other when necessary. However, if one is incapable of offering care at the time, they might ask their daughter to take on the role of caregiver. If the daughter has had a long-term and tense relationship with one or other parent, she might find the role very difficult as she would be more likely to be conscripted out of familial duty.

Younger families that have expectations for the future can have their hopes and dreams come crashing down. Their roles change from an adult-to-adult interaction between each other to an interaction where one party is dependent and the other party is the caregiver. Their hopes have been transgressed.[6]

The life stage of families plays a very significant role in the way that caregiving is experienced. Two family therapists developed a chart showing what people generally do over time or during their life.[7] The six stages of life cycle tasks they categorised appear in Table 9.1.

When there is an interruption to these stages major adjustments need to happen, as one person will often need to straddle their own life stage development and perhaps that of one's parent or child or both. When there is an incompletion of or interruption to a life stage without an understanding or choice about the matter, it may often result in unresolved grief issues at a later stage.

The average age of a carer in Europe is between forty-five and sixty years of age. Both men and women provide care but, not surprisingly, women dominate. Female carers are now much more likely to be in the workforce than were their past counterparts. Most carers have children not yet completely launched into independent living. Today many of the women who care are single parents as well. These women have competing and multifaceted responsibilities.

The family's beliefs about the care of an ageing or ill parent also has consequences. If the belief that 'we care for our own' is strongly held by the family, this may put the carer in an invidious situation.

Table 9.1

Family life cycle stages	Emotional process of transition: key principles	Second-order changes in family status required to proceed developmentally
1. Leaving home Single young adults	Accepting emotional and financial responsibility for self	a. Differentiation of self in relation to family of origin b. Development of intimate peer relationships c. Establishment of self re work and financial independence
2. The joining of families through marriage: the new couple	Commitment to new system	a. Formation of marital system b. Realignment of relationships with extended families and friends to include spouse
3. Families with young children	Accepting new members into the system	a. Adjusting marital system to make space for child(ren) b. Joining in childbearing, financial and household tasks c. Realignment of relationships with extended families to include parenting and grandparenting roles
4. Families with adolescents	Increasing flexibility of family boundaries to include children's independence and grandparents' frailties	a. Shifting of parent–child relationships to permit adolescents to move in and out of system b. Refocus on mid-life marital and career issues c. Beginning shift toward joint caring of older generation
5. Launching children and moving on	Accepting a multitude of exits from and entries into the family system	a. Renegotiation of marital system as two people b. Development of adult–adult relationships between grown children and their parents c. Realignment of relationships to include in-laws and grandchildren d. Dealing with disabilities and death of parents (grandparents)
6. Families in later life	Accepting the shifting of generational roles	a. Maintaining own and/or couple functioning and interests in face of physiological decline; exploration of new familial and social role options b. Support for a more central role of middle generation c. Making room in the system for the wisdom and experience of the elderly, supporting the older generation without functioning for them d. Dealing with loss of spouse, siblings and other peers and preparation for own death. Life review and integration

They may want to support the family belief while struggling with the daily challenges presented by caring for the person with dementia, which is vastly different from that of normal ageing. One of the most challenging aspects of care for a person with dementia is negotiating between the perceived and the actual reality: the person still looks the same but is in fact very different, hence the broader set of adjustments that carers face in the wake of the new level of dependency.[8]

The many faces of caring

Caring always means that one is going to give of one's emotional reserves, being there in a very special way. 'The really tough thing about dementia care is that this is someone you have known in another context, perhaps a really happy marriage, a supportive and nurturing parent, a loving partner and now you have the sense that it is in ruins, and many hopes are not going to come true.'[9] Alternatively, it can bring negative or mixed feelings; people may be caught between what one 'should' do as opposed to what one 'wants' to do. Prior relationships with the person with dementia are significant in terms of how the journey will be experienced for both the carer and the person with dementia. Sometimes it is more helpful if care is relocated outside the family as the tension and stress may be counterproductive for all parties.

Carers often experience overwhelming feelings of being out of control for varying lengths of time. Most will adopt a familiar coping style that has served them in the past in other situations. Others may be totally devastated by the diagnosis, particularly if the person is young and there is no warning of this individual and family catastrophe. The wife of a 46-year-old man with dementia said: 'It is like being in a fog…it has taken me six months to even start to cope. I could not believe that this would happen. He is so young.'

Helping children to cope

Younger people (up to their mid-twenties) require special consideration at the time of diagnosis of a family member as they are in the throes of a multiplicity of development issues of their own. This is a time of physical growth, personal development and conformity, a time for falling in and out of love, leaving home, making career choices and having the desire to fit in with a peer group. Conflicts with parents often occur around this time, as younger people are trying to gain a separate identity from their parents. The additional trials faced when there is a parent or a grandparent diagnosed with dementia can result in both parties feeling a lack of understanding and support.[10]

If the person diagnosed is a parent, the adult children can feel torn between feeling responsible for the parent's care and for the needs of their children. Alternatively if it is a spouse, there is the loss of the partner and the entire attendant issues. The children can either be initially excluded or called upon for support. This support may not be forthcoming as the children struggle to adapt and accept their own loss of a parent. Each member of a family will be in a life cycle of their own that requires constant adaptations to enable people to move to the next stage of life.

The adjustment process

With a progressive illness like dementia, family members will be required to make continual adaptation and role changes if the primary caregiver is to be appropriately supported. In the early stages families may be caught between the desire for intimacy and a pull to let go emotionally from the person with the dementia. The future expectation of loss can make it very hard for family members to keep a balanced perspective. Outsiders and the person with dementia can view emotional responses to the diagnosis by the family as inappropriate. While the person with dementia will be seeking support as they struggle to survive with their cognitive impairment and their own gradual loss of identity.

Family adaptation to loss involves shared grieving and reorganisation of the family relationship. When the patient and or the family hide knowledge of the illness and try to protect their own and each other's feelings, communication barriers create distance and misunderstanding.[11]

One carer shares her experience of part of her adaptation process from being in the role of a wife to the role of a carer:

> When you first find out, it is your own kind of psychological adjustment of acceptance and it takes quite a while. It would be nice to be able to suddenly switch, but it is just that slow constant adjustment to things. This is hard at any time. You need to recognise that it is very difficult to always have to take on board that this is happening all around you.

Often there is a problem in the relationship that is attributed to a lack of initiative by the undiagnosed person. What looks like a marital problem at first may be a disguised change of role from that of a partner to carer.

> A lot of things that were happening in our relationship breakdown were due to John not initiating anything or contributing to the relationship. He just wanted me to cook a meal for him at night, have somewhere to put his head down and go and play bowls all the time.

One young wife makes the painful realisation that her husband would never work again. She lives as a couple, but her role has changed to that of a single person and single parent.

> When I realised that he would never work again I had to find out exactly where I was placed and how the children were placed. I would come home after a nine-hour day. He would not ask me how my day was, he never mentioned Mum's death, it means nothing. It can't. There is a lack of empathy, it's heartbreaking. I tried to get a will written and because he has no insight he couldn't see the point. It's so hard because it should be so normal. I do try

and take the children out hill walking. But it is hard for me because I don't necessarily want to go hill walking…I've got to take them out and do something with them but some Saturdays I just don't want to have to do that. I work five days a week and because he does not drive any more everything is foisted back on me…we do not go out as a couple any more.

Not only are roles reversed within the family home—the ripple effects reach into the realms of sociability, coupleship and adult recreation.

Keeping secrets

Past experience affects what people do in the early stages. Couples make decisions based on many things, one of the most common decisions being that their partner will not be treated differently to other people. One particular woman moved into the role of protector, as her experiences in life had demonstrated that people with mental illness or cognitive impairment were not given equal privileges. This was such a strong belief for her and her husband that she excluded all the adult children in the first few years.

The kids thought that he had depression, but when we received the diagnosis we discussed the issue of who to tell. It was horrible, I just wanted to protect him, and I wanted to cover it up. I did that and it was incredibly hard. We were a blended family and we decided that we would not tell anyone. We did not tell the children (all in their early to mid-twenties). That decision was based on the concern that they and others would treat him differently, like he was stupid. He had that idea from thirty years' experience of dealing with people who fit into some category of mental disability. We wanted things to stay the same.

Denial

Denial is a reaction to the situation. It is not so much about a person's identity or role reversal; it is one way in which people take the necessary time to adjust to the changes that occur within the family. One father recalls that:

> Our sons did not react at first, they were upset but they didn't really believe it. They disappeared and got on with their lives. They only saw her for a short while every few weeks or so. Suddenly the enormity of the situation hit them. One boy is in counselling to help him cope and the other one just cries from time to time. It's unimaginably tough.

Anger

All reactions are individual ways in which families try to adapt to the uninvited changes that are occurring amidst their ranks.

> Our son was about eighteen and for the time before the diagnosis he appeared to have internalised it all. When his dad was finally diagnosed he lost the plot. He was so angry no one could get near him. His sister was in total denial. She behaved as if nothing was wrong.

> I was so angry. I behaved in a manner that was not acceptable but I could not stop. You can't get angry with the person, but you can get angry and ask, 'Why aren't they healthy now, how dare they get sick,' which is completely out of their control and you know that, but it does not stop [your] anger at life. You cope on the outside but on the inside you are going ballistic.

Escaping

Some people will 'escape', either from the family or the situation, while they make adjustment to the situation.

> I had not finished my degree and when I heard the diagnosis I ran away to America for eighteen months. It is a hell of a lot easier not being close to what is going on. I talked to Dad on the phone after he was diagnosed. I couldn't handle it face to face.

After the diagnosis we were told to keep things stable. We laughed and said we didn't think we would do that. I took a job over-seas and was skipping around the countryside and he was back in the hotel. We were very safe in Vietnam. They were very gentle and accepting people.

Fear of inheriting the disease

Some people are still convinced that dementia is a contagious disease.

My son took the diagnosis terribly. I don't think that he has allowed himself to see it objectively—he was so isolated and angry. He was frightened of getting this disease.

Hardship

The people interviewed for this book came from all walks of life and their ages ranged between ten and eighty years of age. One young parent interviewed said she felt that there were too many 'bows' on books about Alzheimer's disease, meaning they did not touch upon the basic hardships for young parent carers with children.

For example: adapting to a role reversal; becoming a single parent operationally while still categorised as married; losing a compan-ion for social occasions; being asked what is the name of that restaurant every five minutes, what is the name of that doctor?; my husband answering the phone and not taking messages; [feel-ing like I am] being shadowed all the time; not being able to go to the toilet or take a shower… or go shopping alone to get some head space; having friends not even ask about you, or him any more, [because they] cannot cope with their feelings of powerless-ness; coping with the issues around children's education and the snob factor inherent in the school playground when a father is no longer employed; the silent scream of 'I don't want to do this bloody, fucking caring job. I want my life back, I don't want to have to explain everything fifty times.' The rage, the exhaustion, isolation and the aloneness. Dementia invades every fibre of your

life. Making a peanut butter sandwich becomes a production.
Other times I know that this will pass but today it feels like hell.

Financial adjustments

Most people live up to or beyond their generated income. When someone loses their salary, the effects are absorbed primarily within the family. Other people may know about it, but the fact remains that it is the family who will bear the brunt of the loss. This changes what the family can and cannot do. The costs involved in getting a diagnosis, and the loss of income after a diagnosis, are significant. There is also very little information available about financial options, which suggests that public awareness is extremely limited.

The effect on ten families

Family carers in Australia conducted an excellent study of ten families that had a person with 'younger onset dementia', that is, onset before sixty-five years of age. They clearly identified that 'families caring for people with early onset dementia carried enormous financial burden for many years…the duration of the pre-diagnosis period was critical in determining what reserve funds were available to face the long haul after diagnosis'.[12]

Prior to diagnosis, combined family incomes ranged from $50 000 or $60 000 to greater than $100 000 per annum. This was the baseline for these families up to the time that significant memory loss or other changes were noticed.

The length of time prior to diagnosis fell between three and seven years. It was during this time that the family felt that something was different or was amiss. Some families were in successful businesses that collapsed and were non-recoverable.

In financial terms we are much worse off. My wife works full-
time now. We had to close our company down because I was

responsible for the major business part of it, and if I made a mistake we could have lost everything.

Another person with younger onset dementia was having difficulty with his business and was incapable of briefing the lawyer on the facts required to defend his court case. His wife stepped in and effectively briefed the lawyer, who defended the case successfully.

Another person was made redundant: she had the double disadvantage of not being able to access a disability pension under the company's superannuation scheme, as the reason given for her retrenchment was that she was unable to cope with the new technology installed at work.

When a diagnosis was made, most of the families had already incurred significant cost in medical expenses for testing, including the neuropsychological testing and brain scans. Some families paid up to $3000 prior to the medical funds reimbursements available to them. Motor vehicle accidents and attendant costs prior to the time of diagnosis also drained families' savings, as some people were unable to pay for car insurance when the breadwinner had lost his/her job. Extra costs, combined with the primary loss of income for the family, impacted on all aspects of the families' lives, even the children's education.

Medications were another significant cost. As these people were under the age of sixty-five (one person was only in their thirties), they had no senior pharmaceutical benefits. The cost of anti-dementia drugs alone ranged from $50 to $240 per month at that time, which did not include other non-prescription medications. Changes to the home, and physical aids, community transport and day care facilities were all paid for from family savings.

Services and financial aid

Services for people with dementia over the age of sixty-five years have been in existence for the past fifteen years and, while they require revision, an inequity exists for younger people, who are estimated to make up 10 per cent of the total of patients diagnosed with some form of dementia. Governments are still encouraging families to keep people with dementia at home, but younger people with families are often at their most difficult time in financial terms, with children not yet launched, mortgages not paid in full, and a person with dementia who requires support, supervision and care twenty-four hours per day. This is not about more needs due to age but about awareness in the wider community as to the emotional and financial difficulties for these families.

Each family is unique and will manage things differently. The common denominator is the need for adaptation to financial losses and major life changes. The crippling costs and financial hardship for the duration of the years ahead need to be looked at by policy-makers so they can provide support for younger families where dementia occurs. There are at present no younger-people-specific policies that adequately address these hidden costs.

Grief and loss

The diagnosis of dementia of a family member is inextricably linked with some form of loss and grief. What exactly is grief? It is the emotional reaction to loss. Losses we recognise are divorce, family fragmentation after divorce, end of a friendship, giving up a child for adoption or losing a pet. All of these situations involve loss but do not involve death. Other losses include loss of income, loss of a promotion, family relocation, immigration, marriage of a child, all of which result in some form of grief. This does not mean that the actual person is lost, but the attachment that we had to something or someone has changed.

Grief may be experienced as a sudden catastrophic reaction or it may come in waves that make a person feel as if they are drowning and have to struggle to the surface gasping for air. The most common symptoms of grief are:

- **Feelings**, such as sadness, anger, guilt, reproach, anxiety, loneliness, fatigue, helplessness, shock, yearning and numbness.
- **Physical sensations**, such as hollowness in the stomach, tightness in the chest and throat, oversensitivity to noise, a sense of depersonalisation, shortness of breath, muscle weakness, lack of energy and dry mouth.
- **Cognitions**, such as disbelief, confusion, pre-occupation, sense of presence and hallucinations.
- **Behaviours**, such as sleep and appetite disturbances, absent-minded behaviour, social withdrawal, searching and calling out, sighing, restless overactivity, crying, visiting places or objects that were memorable, the use of drugs and alcohol to reduce the pain.[13]

Anticipatory grief

'Anticipatory grief' is a phrase that is used to describe a very complicated phenomenon that occurs when there is an opportunity to anticipate the death of a loved one or of oneself.[14] An example would be when there is a serious disease and the doctor has given an estimated length of time that a person could be expected to live. When a person is diagnosed with dementia there is a generalised expectancy of life depending on the type of dementia and the age of diagnosis. Many people collapse at the time of diagnosis and move in and out of thoughts and feelings about the loss of the person, although it may be many years away in reality.

This anticipatory grief is often occurring at the same time as people are adapting with the subtle form of 'change' in the person with memory problems. There may be financial losses, and there may be a relocation of homes for many people as an attempt to either find employment, or to move to more suitable accommodation.

Relocation

There is no research that supports the notion that a smaller dwelling improves the quality of a person's life. Many people that I have spoken to have a deep sense of regret that they have lost space for a library, a garden, a pet or a place down the back yard in which to tinker around. A retired minister said:

> *Every day I rage on the inside at my stupidity at agreeing to come and live in this sterile butter box. I have lost thousands of treasured books and papers because they don't fit in—people do not notice that I don't fit in.*

Relocation can create many unanticipated losses that appear inconsequential at first, such as the loss of one's doctor, dentist, butcher, grocer, neighbours, friends, church and a sense of belonging to a community. Also, loss of privacy and loss of personal space might occur. New does not always mean better.[15]

Working towards hope

'In the factory we make cosmetics, in the store we sell hope.'[16] Grief can be likened to a long dark tunnel we must enter so that we can come out the other end to reach the radiant sunshine again.[17]

The heroine asks her uncle, 'What does one do when the sun of one's happiness is set?' He answers, 'After a time, one lights a candle called patience and guides one's footsteps by that—remembering that you are not alone. More than half of the noblest men and women you meet carry such candles.'[18]

When processing or living through grief it is often believed or feared that a person's life will be forever diminished in some way—that their life will be permanently altered for the worst. This is a natural reaction to a loss or anticipated loss and demands the application of generous amounts of imagination to resolve.

At the tunnel opening you have three choices: to pretend that the loss is not occurring; to acknowledge the loss is occurring or has happened but deny its importance to you; or to accept the loss and begin to work through the grief.[19] The third choice allows you to step into the tunnel and see the tiny star-like light that glimmers microscopically at the end. You may feel the fear, but you keep taking one step at a time and watch the point of light grow larger.

Taking that first step into the tunnel does not have to be a solo journey; you have the option of taking another safe person with you, spiritually or metaphorically, via a counsellor, a minister, priest or rabbi—someone that you trust and has the ability to metaphorically 'hold' you as you work through your fears. A professional person outside the family has the capacity to walk the distance with you and not feel inadequate or powerless when they observe your grief. People close to us often feel exhausted by the feeling that they cannot make us 'feel better'. The uncontained emotionality caused by grief begins to go around in circles bouncing off old wounds that have gone unattended as people have got on with their lives. Your grief is authentically yours and needs to be experienced in a safe and appropriate place. It is an invaluable life experience and requires the utmost respect without judgment or trivialisation.

The grieving process can involve emotions that will swing all over the place like a barometer in a cyclone—sunshine and suffocating heat one moment suddenly followed by torrential rain so heavy and blinding that you cannot see two metres in front of you; wind velocity screaming at a pitch that stops conversations, leaving you only with inadequate hand signals to convey your ineptness against the forces of nature. Such can be the emotional state of grief.

This state is frightening when you are in it but it is also the place that we all go to at some point in our lives and is the starting point for recovery. Feelings of despair and hopelessness frequently go hand in hand with grief. It first needs to be experienced, then understood. We can then begin to detach from an imagined future and surrender our plans. Hope feels lost, but it has only been hidden behind a dense black cloud until the atmospheric conditions allow it to move on and reveal a changed situation.

Accepting loss and coping with grief

There is no set time in which to reinvest in the future, to re-engage with the sense of purpose and hope. Change is not easy for many reasons; it means giving up the comfort of the familiar, having to take a risk, a gamble on something that is uncertain and unpredictable, an unknown for an unknown amount and length of time.

Hope and surrender

This is not a well-defined path and tends to be seen retrospectively. People are often hazy historians when trying to recall exactly when they started to feel better about themselves. Shedding the skin of a past way of being can initially appear demoralising; however, if you have chosen to move through the tunnel you slowly come to the realisation that things will never be the same again. Implanted within this realisation is another set of opportunities and realignment with the emotion of hope. Hope is the essential ingredient of life and projects our dreams and wishes into the future in a positive way. It is the lighthouse, the torch, the dream. It keeps us having something to achieve, to strive for, to believe in.

Hope and purpose are different for each person in the family depending on where they are in their life. However, hope can neutralise anxiety, soothe your fears and create a positive attitude towards life. Hope looks to the next step, whatever form the step may take. Hope has been described as being the fundamental knowledge and feeling that there is a way out of difficulty, that things can work out, that we as human persons can somehow handle and manage internal and external reality, that there are 'solutions' in the most ordinary biological and physiological sense of the word.[20]

It is not necessarily the object of hope that we may have chosen, such as a new home, a child or a new car; rather, it is the feeling that comes with hope. When we temporarily lose hope in something or someone outside of ourselves it can raise the question, 'What do I believe in? What do I stand for in life? What is my real purpose?'

These thoughts may be fleeting and can quickly pass away, but they have been registered both on a conscious and unconscious level and can be retrieved later for closer inspection and development, when the time is right. It is only when our security is challenged or our lives dramatically changed that we look for solace and meaning in our lives. Dreams and wishes are suspended, supplanted by a fear of the unknown. What you can do during this time is bring your attention right into the present time, right now. Look for things that are achievable and realistic. If this seems difficult, test your memory by trying to recall exactly what you were worrying about on this day one year ago? A year ago may seem like another lifetime, but those previous issues have been superseded by the changes that are occurring in your life now. And just as you have survived to tell the story, you will survive this journey also.

To sustain a hopeful stance takes courage and inner strength, but doing so will provide you with an open attitude that allows opportunities to present themselves on your doorstep, offering you choices previously not considered. Everyone likes to have control of their lives, and when your sense of control is taken away for whatever reason it hurts, and you want to regain a sense of control as soon as possible. You want to feel safe, achieve some sense of personal meaning about what is happening around you, and perpetuate your desire for freedom from adversity.

10 The family system

When we try and pick out anything by itself, we find it hitched to everything else in the universe.

John Muir

FAMILIES CAN BE A RICH SOURCE OF SUPPORT FOR A PERSON diagnosed with a dementing illness, as they hold the historical knowledge of who the person was prior to the changes that occur slowly over the years following the diagnosis. Families have knowledge about what has happened or does happen both within and between people in the family. People outside of the family generally have only a one-dimensional view, and do not know the complexities of the interactions that occur between family members and the person with the dementing illness.

In the past, psychotherapy worked hard to keep individuals separate from their families as if the patient arrived on the therapist's doorstep without any internal or external experiences gained from their family of origin. The notion at the time was that that person's pathology was held within them or that they were in some way responsible for what was happening. Slowly the light began to dawn on the therapists that patients usually had a family somewhere, and the family was eventually brought into the picture. The focus then changed from the individual (with the problem) to include the system or (family) from which the person came. The *systemic viewpoint* emerged as a more realistic one in its recognition that many forces, both within and between people, shape the life experience of the person. Pioneering family therapists such as Murray Bowen, Virginia Satir, Carl Whittaker, Jay Hayley, and Salvadore Minuchin did ground-breaking work with families. Later, as family therapy spread to include medical illness, it seemed unreasonable just to provide treatment of a disease without taking into account other variables. Just treating the disease without including the whole person is no longer considered viable in general medical practice.[1]

In essence the term *systemic* involves thinking about families as multiple, interrelated components that make up a whole, and each part of the system directly or indirectly affects every other part of the system. No one is fully separate from the larger system of which they are a part, even if they live in another town or country.

On a personal level one can think about the various components of their life such as occupation, hobbies, relationships, interests. Who is important in your life and why? What type of work do you do? What do you do for recreation and why? What do you believe in? How much education did you formally receive from your family? How much education have you perused in later life and what was the reason for this? Where do you live? What kind of environment do you live in? What sustains you? What did your family value? Where did you fit in the family? What were your family mottos? What caused conflict in your family? Who was the closest to whom and why was this so? How were solutions to problems managed? What was the political climate that you grew up in? What soothes you? Who are you closest to in your own family?

The purpose of this exercise is to demonstrate that you are much more than a name. You as an individual have had millions of experiences that shape the way you think and behave. If you focus on only one aspect of yourself (say, where you now live) you lose the bigger picture about how you have arrived at a certain place in your life. Similarly, if you select one person from a family to focus upon you can miss important facts and experiences that affect the way they behave or operate both publicly and privately. All the members of a family (or system) have an effect upon each other and their view of the world. Even family members who do not speak to each other or are dead all have a place or role in the family. If one part of the system is traumatised by some life event, then all the other members will be affected to a greater or lesser degree.

Shared experiences in a family's history will create triggers or flags. Also, every member of a family will respond to different situations in different ways as they have both the family experiences and their own personal ones.

Rather than thinking along the lines of cause and effect family therapists see family interactions as circular, which suggests there is a mutual influence on events such as when A does this then B does that. This 'dance' can very soon become one of blame or 'Look what you have done to me'. This is unhelpful when a family member is hurting and is exhausted by trying to cope with the events that occur following the diagnosis of a dementing illness.

The commercial jingle 'this goes with that' used to sell the new season's outfits is an excellent example of a family system. When the outfit is first modelled the marketing people attempt to persuade the buyers that this 'outfit' has a 'must have' identity. This new style may be worn by day, to business, evening, country and beach events and so forth. The marketers have done their job when the product is sold and worn like a badge of honour, heralding the fact that the wearer is in fashion or up to date. The young girls may look similar in the new look but there is much more underneath.

The outfit does not depict the threads in each garment, where the fabric was made, who did the sewing or how many hands the garment went through while being made. It does not depict the trucks or docks, staff, electronic security machines or the stands that have been moved around the shop. Each new manager to a store will automatically change the clothes around or be part of a publicity campaign created to sell the product. The retailers have done their job by selling the illusion of leisure. If there is a glitch in the system, of some of its thousands of components, the company loses a lot of money. If the salesperson was blamed for poor sales without investigating all the other points along the journey, then all that would happen would be that the salesperson could lose their job and the problem is only temporarily solved—it will resurface again.

In real life a family glitch can result in emotional pain, family cut-offs and a sick and dysfunctional family. As the situation gets more rigidly entrenched there is little joy within the family and solutions can appear light years away.

Family systemic therapy aims to understand how the problem is being maintained and whose needs are being met either negatively or positively. Embedded in the problem there is always the answer to another riddle.

11 Caring for the carer

CARERS ARE PEOPLE WHO AT SOME TIME MAY BE REQUIRED TO do things that would normally be classified as socially abnormal by other people; for example, a daughter-in-law may be required to shower her father-in-law. This may not be a regular occurrence but, in terms of being a carer, it may be necessary.

At the onset of the disease carers experience a nearly vertical learning curve as they try to live with changes such as the constant repetitive questions that are part of the problem caused by memory impairment. It is not unusual for people to use communication methods that are not helpful, which will only cause themselves and the person with early stage dementia to feel even more powerless and angry. It bears a stark resemblance to the way people raise their voice in an attempt to have non-English speaking background people understand English, or the expectation that a blind person will understand what a sighted person is seeing. This is the genesis of carer distress: they do not know what to do, or how to do it. However, this does not mean that they are unwilling to learn. One carer said:

I went along with him to all the appointments, in fact I arranged all the appointments. The only recognition that I received was from the receptionist, who offered me some choice about his next appointment in six months time. When we arrived home, nothing had changed for me except that I knew that he had Alzheimer's disease. I had known something was wrong for months, as I had been filling in the gaps and spaces for him. I sat down and cried my heart out while he went off to watch the news on the TV.

In order to achieve caring effectively and with the least amount of harm to oneself and the person being cared for, it is important to see caring as a defined role and not a redefinition of self. Carers are often thought of as some homogeneous group of people who by choice or circumstance provide care for another person. This global representation of a carer is limited in that it depersonalises the individual who is placed under the label of being 'a carer'.

My concern is that if the individual needs of the carer go unacknowledged and unsupported, where do these 'needs' go? In a perfect world they could be absorbed by a caring, nurturing family and a supportive network of friends. For some people these situations are far from perfect, or are non-existent at the outset (around the time of diagnosis) because it is commonly thought that carers do not need support in the early stages or that carers do not tell others for fear of being stigmatised. However, support is most needed at the outset because it lays the groundwork for the later stages and carers then know that they are not alone. This single act can lay foundations for building trust and confidence for the whole journey and provide a safety net in the present and in the future.

It is easier to contact a person in whom you have confidence or with whom you have had previous contact than it is to reach out to a stranger when anxiety and stress are high.

In the early stages of dementia people do not need a 'carer' in the formal sense of doing things, such as being responsible or taking over roles that were previously held by the person with dementia. However, there is a change in the level of awareness about the other person as memory, mood or personality changes require adaptations by the family, even if they are subtle.

People who become carers have their own personal agendas, attitudes and beliefs about care, life histories, needs and wants, family situations, occupational dilemmas and differences in physical and mental health status, all of which contribute to the way that care is delivered. Primary caregivers stress is well researched; it has been reported[1] that 'dementia caregivers have worse health, a poorer immunological response and a higher use of drugs such as tranquillisers, sleeping pills and alcohol'. As opposed to normal reactions of stress, carer distress is very complex and subjective. Carers often complain of the physical and psychological symptoms of clinical depression; these treatable features may be overlooked if designated collectively to the label of carer burden or carer stress by health professionals.

The operative words here are complex and subjective. If complex and subjective needs are not allowed to be tabled and are not addressed in a safe, supportive environment, they will become problematical. Most literature refers to the carer as the person who does things for another, and the reciprocal loop of what the carer unconsciously or inadvertently imposes on the person with dementia is rarely discussed. The question that this poses is: 'Are all carers angels?', or are they just like the rest of us fallible human beings that have experienced hurts and joys to a greater or lesser extent in their life?

The fact that some carers do undoubtedly become depressed, hurt, exhausted and unfortunately forgotten by some people who they thought would be there for them is indisputable, but do the unmet needs of carers impact upon the person with dementia? If so, where is the voice of the person with dementia when their speech and thought patterns are reduced? Perhaps the only avenue left for them is their behaviour, which is often seen as the problem.

A world specialist in dementia, Tom Kitwood, proposes that carers need to rework their relationship with the person who has dementia. By the term rework he means:

> *A relationship builds up a lot of mutual expectations—each person expects their needs to be met by the other. If a carer is still expecting their needs to be met in the relationship (as time goes by) then most certainly it is going to be deeply disappointing. But if they can let go and start seeing and handling the relationship in a radical new way, then often it turns out to be more OK than what we might have expected.*[2]

This reworking of a previously good relationship provides many challenges in terms of gaining a different perspective of the previously known relationship and drawing on inner strengths perhaps previously not required to the same level. However, if the relationship has a lot of unresolved issues and was not particularly close for many reasons, it is either a time to try and resolve some of the past hurts or to look outside the relationship for alternative ways to provide care. If a husband or wife had not felt valued or respected in the marriage and is now expected to be a carer, this is very difficult—as it is for the child who never felt special or cared for by the parent and is now expected to become the carer. People who never chose the task of caring are often personally and privately resentful of having to be in a role for which they perceive they have no predisposition. Yet, because they are the spouse or other family member they cannot see any options, especially if they are women.

Caring for the caregiver

Couple counselling has proven to be helpful to people in the early stages of dementia to assist with the adaptations that are required within the relationship, and to help each individual cope with their own personal issues.[3] Research in this area has been sparse, but there are some very good studies and more in the making. One study in particular consisted of structured counselling sessions for caregivers at the beginning of the treatment process—two with the primary caregiver and four with the family. Primary caregivers were asked to participate in a weekly support group and ongoing counselling was provided at the request of the carer on an ad hoc basis. The findings of this program, which lasted for a couple of years, concluded that people in the early to middle stages of dementia, in particular, did not need admission to a nursing home until much later as the carers were able to cope at home longer than usual.

In particular, carers need to be taught not to take the patient's behaviour personally, which is much easier said than done. It often requires formal psychotherapy and intervention with the carer.

Why is it all so personal?

Why do carers often take the person with dementia's behaviour so personally? If they are a family member there is a long history involved, both conscious and unconscious. One theory suggests that generally mothers set a strong foundation for future relations. Knowing that all of our earliest experiences with our parents become part of our living story and affect our present relationships is an important concept. An example of this would be when some event occurs and we have very strong reactions to the event that when looked at retrospectively seem disproportionate to the event.

This idea is further suggested: 'there's no such thing as marriage, merely two scapegoats sent out by their families to perpetuate themselves'. Soo Borson, an Associate Professor of Psychiatry was making an understatement when she suggested that carers try to not take the person with dementia's behaviour personally. She further posed that carers need to be viewed as patients as they often require treatment for depression, chronic stress responses and anger, as well as grief, anticipatory grief, disenfranchised grief and ambiguous loss.

On the taking it personally issue, relationships are very complex issues with multiple levels of meaning. Every nuance has a different interpretation by someone in the family, so it is important to learn ways to depersonalise the behaviour of the person with dementia and not the person themselves. That is the crux of the matter.

Adjustment disorders

An unexpected diagnosis of dementia is a traumatic event, often leaving the family so traumatised that they become what appears to be dysfunctional for an indefinite length of time. The family is really not dysfunctional but they can look dysfunctional, exhibiting readily diagnosed symptoms of adjustment disorders such as depression, anxiety, stress, somatic illnesses or a mixture of anxiety and depression. It is important that the family does not get labelled as dysfunctional because of an initial inability to cope with a major life stressor. Normal grief is not considered an adjustment disorder.

The symptoms of stress normally include hopelessness, sadness, crying, anxiety, worry, headaches, withdrawal, reckless driving, fighting in the family, other destructive acts and disturbances in sleep patterns.

Treatment

Psychotherapy is the treatment of choice for adjustment disorders, as the problem is caused by a very understandable reaction to a specific stress. Family or couple therapy is the preferred treatment and will focus on issues such as:

- Understanding the meaning of the diagnosis of dementia to individual family members.
- Understanding how the diagnosis has affected their lives.
- Developing coping skills.

- Discussing aspects of dementia and the meaning of it for them.
- Normalising their reactions after the meaning of the adjustment symptoms have been clarified with them.
- Empowering them with ways to cope by building a resourceful network.

Most people recover completely if they have had no previous history of mental health problems. Medication is not usually used except for a few days or weeks of anti-anxiety drugs to control anxiety or sleeping problems.

Depression in carers

Depression used to be considered as a failure to cope or the sign of a person lacking sufficient intestinal fortitude—all negative connotations about one's personhood with the result that many people suffered quietly and for a long time. Depression was likened to a contagious mental illness. Now the pendulum has swung the other way and depression is acknowledged as the fourth most common problem treated by general practioners. Prescriptions for anti-depression drugs have soared by 60 per cent, and it is thought that this increase is a reflection of less hesitancy by GPs to record this diagnosis.[4]

There are various forms of depression. Some people may only experience one episode of depression in their whole life but others may have some recurrences. Some people may have a depressive episode for no apparent reason, while for others it can be associated with a life situation or stress. Just like dementia, depression is a word, and while it may be of some assistance to know that it is a condition that is treatable with medication, that does not help us to understand why we have these feelings. Professionals in this field have written about breaking the patterns of depression, exposing the belief that life is all about the interpretation of how you see things, how you make meaning of your life.[5] Each day you continually explain things to yourself, about yourself and about events in the world around you. Each person develops a style of explaining things to self; this is called your explanatory style and it has a huge role in how you feel.

Imagine that you had been caring for your father, who had been a wonderful parent, and since he had developed dementia you had increased your vigilance regarding his whereabouts. He was only in the early to moderate stage and was physically fit but tended to go walkabout, and there had been a couple of occasions where the police were requested to assist in finding him. Your friends knew about his behaviour and, regardless of this, made a genuine offer to 'care' for him while you took some time out.

Self-talk could go something like this: 'These people are really genuine and I really value their support.' You perhaps feel warm and safe. If then you think, 'But what if he is difficult and runs away and spoils their evening while I am out enjoying myself,' he could become an imposition and you could naturally become ambivalent about leaving him. Then you think, 'He really is my responsibility. He was always there for me as a child, and now I should be there for him.' You could start to feel guilty or responsible and that you should keep it in the family, and you remember that you are the only family that he has. The feeling of guilt resurfaces between your need to take care of yourself and the need to let go and trust someone else to support you.

This is an example of how what we say to ourselves has a direct consequence on how we feel about a situation. Ambivalence or conflicting emotions leave us stuck and make it difficult to move in any direction. In this situation many carers will tend to say, 'Oh! Thank you very much but I am really all right at the moment. But I will definitely call on you at some other time.' Underneath your behaviour is a thinking pattern that is formed by a whole set of beliefs that you just see as part of who you are. And as scenarios similar to the one mentioned here are repeated, people may stop offering their help and they really start to believe that you are okay, and are coping just fine.

On the one hand, the recounting of events around caring sound exhausting, but when support is offered it is declined. If the carer's pattern of thinking is ambiguous it is a calling card for depression. Everyone carries a list of injunctions imposed upon them long before they ever had a person with dementia in their lives, and these injunctions need to be explored because without making meaning of your behaviour you will tend to repeat it and become isolated, distressed and depressed. Anti-depressant medication can stabilise your mood, but it does not change the situation until you can understand what is happening to you on the inside and make some sense out of it. This can be done more quickly with a trained facilitator or counsellor who can help you understand your responses. It's a bit like the riddle: 'How do you eat an elephant? A mouthful at a time.'

Stress—what it actually is

When you fall in love you can become vulnerable and hypersensitive, excitable, energised and, to onlookers, you could also be viewed as slightly silly. Stress can have similar feelings without the accompanying smile and abundance of unlimited joy. Both love and stress are in the eyes of the beholder; what is stressful to one person will not necessarily affect another person in the same way.

Stress is a fairly new word, in that it was not used a great deal prior to the 1980s. It is yet another word that is universally used but the actual meaning is open to interpretation, as it is mostly a subjective experience that brings with it ambiguity. It is not an illness. Rather, it could be seen as a 'process', with its duration and depth relieved or worsened by the individual circumstance.

When you become a carer you will move from one position in life to another. This adaptation may be laden with stressors such as external factors, job, house move, family, legal and financial issues, people, further medical investigations, doctor's appointments and your state of physical health. On the inside will be variable degrees of anxiety, anger and fatigue, all of which have to be dealt with. Depending on your situation, the duration of the stress will be influenced by the support you receive, your beliefs about illness, your attitude to the diagnosis, your past history of coping and adaptability, your age and that of your family, your expectations about life and how you adapt to change.

Stress can be viewed as a process that is initiated when demands exceed readily available resources. Uninvited change, as with the diagnosis of dementia, can cause a catastrophic reaction in some people that can take some time to resolve. However some will systematically look for solutions to life issues and work through them one at a time. They will put up their hand for assistance at the outset and will be offered support to attend to those life issues that will be affected by the diagnosis. Stress, therefore, is not the same for each person and each situation needs to be assessed individually.

Stress and anxiety can look very similar. Symptomatic relief can be achieved by medication but the underlying situation and the meaning of the stressors to the individual need to be partially if not fully understood in order to assist the carer to move to a more resilient position. Poet, artist and philosopher Kahlil Gibran published his views on sorrow and joy in this way:

> Joy is your sorrow unmasked.
> And the selfsame well from which your laughter rises was often times filled with your tears.
> The deeper that sorrow carves into your being the more joy you can contain.
> Is not the cup that holds your wine the very cup that was burned in the potter's oven?
> And is not the lute that soothes your spirit the very wood that was hollowed with knives?

When you are joyous, look deep into your heart and you shall find it is not only that which has given you sorrow that is giving you joy.

When you are sorrowful, look again in your heart and you shall see that in truth you are weeping for that which has been your delight.

Verily you are suspended like scales between your sorrow and your joy.

Only when you are empty are you at a standstill and balanced.

When the treasure-keeper lifts you to weight his gold and silver, needs must your joy or your sorrow rise and fall.[6]

12 Hidden loss

THERE ARE MANY RESPONSES TO THE DIAGNOSIS OF DEMENTIA, from catastrophic disbelief to philosophical acceptance of life's events. Irrespective of the reaction, there will be the loss of the person as they had previously been known and people will experience some form of grief. There may also be anticipatory grief (discussed in Chapter 9), which arises when there is an opportunity to anticipate the loss of a loved one.[1] The impact will affect individuals at every level. Aspects will involve the past that was shared and can never be regained, the present—the losses that occur in terms of diminishing capabilities— and the future, through anticipation of the loneliness and the events that will not be shared. As one wife said:

> When I think of the years my husband has invested in our children's lives, such as their education and sporting activities, I now realise that he will no longer share in the special milestones of life such as graduation, marriage and the births of our grandchildren.

Grief is not restricted to death. Death has social sanction and there are many rituals associated with the loss of a significant person in the family. However, the grief referred to here is deep and long, and there is no ritual. Grief is commonly understood as an emotional reaction to loss. Chapter 2 detailed many reactions to the diagnosis of dementia, reactions that were individual responses to anticipated loss. Some people ran away, cut themselves off, kept the diagnosis secret, felt alienated by the family, became angry, isolated themselves, or realigned with their families of origin when there had been a blended family in place for many years. All these behaviours are the individual's way of trying to adjust to the loss without any social acknowledgment of that loss.

The family is the source from which we learn how to interpret the experiences you meet in your world. They give you cues about appropriate reactions. However, over time, people's lives and world views change from that of the family, hence the different reactions to grief. Some families become closer during uncertain times, while others split apart and begin to fight with each other as yet another way of personally trying to absorb a loss. There is no right way or wrong way.

Ambiguous losses are those that are unclear. Uncertainty is the key element; people are unsure about exactly what is lost or when it will be lost, while friends and social networks may even avoid the same level of interaction with the individual or family because they too are uncomfortable with the uncertainty. Ambiguous losses include peri-natal death, the loss of a lover, AIDS deaths, suicide or murder, divorce, chronic illness, when a child gets involved in drugs, or loss of a pet. There are many such losses that people absorb alone throughout their lives and which are not socially validated, resulting in the griever not being socially recognised. This list includes the losses associated with Alzheimer's disease and other dementing illnesses, especially when the person suffering from dementia can no longer identify a family member. The carer experiences ambiguous loss, living each day with uncertainty. This uncertainty is further increased when people speak about the person with dementia in their presence, as if they were not there. What is seen as carer burnout could, in fact, be unrecognised ambiguous loss.

Families with Alzheimer's were researched as recently as 2000 and it was found that the severity of the patients' dementia bore no relationship to the extent of their caregivers' depressive symptoms. Rather, it was the degree to which the family caregivers saw the person with dementia as absent or present that strongly predicted their depressive symptoms.

Dr P. Boss was involved in a research project concerning the families of pilots declared missing in action in Vietnam and Cambodia.[2] It was when she was interviewing the wives of the missing pilots that she first 'learned the power of ambiguity in complicating loss'. These women lived with the loss of their husbands on a daily and yearly basis, and no information was forthcoming. There was no official verification that anything had been lost. Boss is of the opinion that of all 'losses experienced in personal relationships, ambiguous loss is the most devastating because it remains unclear and indeterminate'.

The greater the degree of ambiguity surrounding one's loss the more difficult it is to master one's depression, stress, anxiety and family conflict. This is because of a perpetual feeling of being out of control and unsure. In response to this uncertainty, families will often take action to offset the feelings of hopelessness. Action could be ignoring the person with dementia, avoiding the carer, gaining attention by fighting with other family members, acting up at school, or denying that there is anything wrong.

A further complicating factor occurs when people do not know who is 'psychologically in' and who is 'psychologically out' in the family. This is an important concept. A state in which family members are uncertain in their perceptions of who is 'in or out' of the family and who is performing what roles and tasks within the family is defined as boundary ambiguity. Caregivers experience enormous difficulty because the person with dementia may be physically present but emotionally absent for part of the time—the carer is straddling two realities simultaneously and, not unreasonably, can get emotionally stuck in the uncertainty of their role. Are they still a wife, a partner, a mother?

What is their role? Who is their support? Establishing the family networks and potential support systems available within the family is the beginning of a grounding process that offers something that is real to help the carer move forward.

Routinely, when conducting a family interview I draw a genogram, which is a map of a family represented by circles, squares and different lines. A genogram is like a family tree that shows a family's emotional and biological processes over generations. By using symbols to represent males, females, pregnancies, deaths, marriages, de facto relationships, birth order and many other life cycle events that happen in families, a genogram can also show emotional patterns including conflict, closeness and distance between family members.

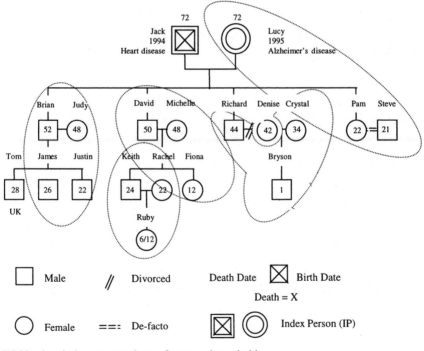

Within the circles are members of current households.

Figure 12.1

A sample genogram

The use of genograms was pioneered by Dr Murray Bowen, a world-famous family therapist who developed the natural systems theory to help understand the lives of people in families according to a universal process. In this universal process, whole and parts of relationships do not go in straight lines but interact with cause and effect with each other because of the interaction between family members over generations. Patterns or ways of behaviour and beliefs are set up and passed down the generations. When people marry, they bring their beliefs and values from their family of origin into the relationship. Often these beliefs lie dormant until there occurs child rearing, financial matters, the need to share basic things like housework, or the need to provide care for a person or a child. This is when differences of opinions or beliefs can occur and need to be resolved if the relationship is to survive.

Families are very dynamic and alter in time. Husband, wife and children living together have been typically defined as the nuclear family, but due to the rising numbers of divorce and second marriages this is no longer the case. Today families are made up of husband, wife and children from current and previous marriages, known as a blended family. Loyalties within families can understandably become fragmented.

Drawing a genogram with the family present helps the family to conceptualise alliances, coalitions and family characteristics, that is, who is closest to whom and often the reasons why. The process of gathering names, dates and marital status provides an opportunity to discuss family traditions and beliefs about dementia.

During this process it becomes clear who is in and who is out of the inner circle with comments such as 'Well, there is Sue and she is in England', or 'Peter is in America'. These comments could indicate that these people were an afterthought or weren't considered to be part of the family because of the geographical distances. Alternatively, one person may live in Ireland but be the family organiser and hold a very definite role even though living in another country. Not all the family members present at the session will agree totally upon who is closest to whom, but they will have a loose agreement or even ambivalence.

Complicating the situation are children from blended families; the divorced parents' relationship, visiting arrangements, occupants of households and for what length of time all constitutes 'the family', but each person will have a different view. Granddaughters can be closer to a grandparent than to one of their own parents—this is not uncommon. Also, the 'inner circle' changes along with life cycle issues. Just because there are six children in a family it does not necessarily mean that there will be someone who will volunteer to be a carer.

Finding out who is willing and available to support the carer is the beginning of change. The family system starts to slowly shift to begin the process of accommodating, in a different way, the position that was held previously by the person with dementia.

Uncertainty and misunderstanding about family roles—who does what, who decides what, when and where—is a very common occurrence, especially when families are under stress. All families have some system within which they operate, and to be effective families need to understand the (unwritten) rules and to agree to abide by them. Without this partial or total understanding of the rules the family cannot move forward to resolve the stress.

If the roles remain unclear the family has boundary ambiguity; without clearly defined boundaries they will collapse under the pressure. Family boundaries cannot be maintained by outsiders—they must be maintained from the inside by you and your family. When there is a clear, healthy family boundary, a major barrier to management and stressful events is overcome. When change occurs in a family, each person needs to know where they or their role ends and the next person's role begins.[3]

The importance of boundaries

Boundaries are invisible lines drawn within and among family members. These form subsystems such as a boy and his dog, a husband

and wife, grandparents, two girls in the family who are very close and share secrets, or even a mother and a child. One family member can belong to a number of subsystems. Part of the therapist's role is to help the family either to strengthen or loosen family boundaries, depending on the situation. For example, if a grandparent ignores the parent's wishes and makes one of the grandchildren more special than the other grandchild, the parental boundary and the sibling subsystem has been unbalanced. This can cause resentment and stress in the family because the grandparent has usurped a parent's power. Boundaries can be clear, rigid or diffuse.

Clear boundaries provide definitive separation between subsystems within a system.

Unclear boundaries. If a father overidentifies (or sees himself as being very similar to his son—on one hand he is a parent, and on the other hand he wants to be the son's best friend), the son will have difficulty responding appropriately. The father wants to be obeyed one minute, and then be his son's buddy the next. In this example the mother is then left out of the picture, because the father has a need to be the boy's best friend. As a parent, he should consult with his wife when it comes to parenting issues. When he steps out of a parenting role, into a buddy role, the child becomes confused, as the boundaries are unclear. A clear boundary needs to be in place for the parents and the child to assume their respective roles. This ensures that the relationships can be healthy and functional.

Diffuse boundaries Problems in families with diffuse boundaries are not contained between the appropriate people, such as between parents. Personal and private issues are spread thoughout the entire family, affecting each member, rather than remaining confined in the subsystem. For example, if there is a problem with the father's work, he could discuss it with his wife until the work situation becomes clearer and they have made some decisions. Or they could discuss the work problem with the pre-teenage children—who in turn could begin to worry unnecessarily about the situation for which they are not responsible. This situation can often be seen as family closeness, but often, it is more about unclear boundaries.

Overinvolvement or overprotectiveness, on the part of the parent with a child, affects both parents and the child's relationship with all the members of the family. A false sense of belonging is gained by sacrificing the child's autonomy or sense of self.

A daughter who has been overinvolved with her mother may have felt close and special as a child but later in life she is not encouraged to have her own life. This can lead to feelings of guilt and being torn between the needs of her own family and the needs of her mother.

Rigid boundaries are boundaries that are relatively impermeable, making it difficult for information to flow between subsystems in a family. This can lead to the family becoming emotionally cut off from each other. There is little opportunity for interaction, the display of feelings or having a sense of belonging. Relationships between family members are weak or non-existent.

Picture this scenario: a father is involved in making his first million dollars, the mother is overinvolved in golf, the son is at university concentrating on becoming an engineer, the twelve-year-old daughter is brought home by the police for being involved in an incident with a stolen car. Years later this daughter can be depicted as the uninvolved child who does not want to be involved in family issues such as dementia.[4] If this lack of involvement by a daughter is taken at face value the origins of the cut-off could easily be misinterpreted in a very negative light, rather than understanding the situation where the daughter was largely ignored as the family were engaged with their own pursuits when she was growing up.

Differentiation

When a person has a low level of differentiation they will be pulled in all directions by the needs of others rather than their own needs. Low levels of differentiation provide a hotbed for breeding feelings of resentment and powerlessness and acts of martyrdom.

It is more likely to be caused by beliefs such as, *look after others before yourself,* handed down intergenerationally as family tenets, and *putting self first is conceited, vain, uncaring and selfish.* It is no wonder that adult carers get caught up in wondering how much care is enough. Where do the boundaries get drawn? How much care *is* enough. How much time do you have? How do you balance your needs against the needs of caring?

Differentiation is the ability to maintain a non-anxious presence in the face of others' anxiety, and is not the same as being uninvolved or indifferent. Differentiation is the ingredient that allows people to be intensely involved without becoming contaminated with other people's anxiety. It prevents the need to withdraw from or interfere with, other people's modus operandi. This lack of reactivity, discomfort or defensiveness affords the carer the opportunity to take care of their own needs first. When we travel on an aircraft and the airline staff is presenting the emergency drill, they say something like 'Mothers should not put the oxygen on the children first. They must put it on themselves so they can help the children.' It seems more natural to put the oxygen on the children first so they will be safe, but in this instance the mother can offer more if she is 'cared' for first.

I cannot fly and hear this oxygen drill without being reminded of the need for self-differentiation. This is not a state that comes easily to most people; it requires revisiting many times, even on a daily basis. This is not about lack of love for the other person, it is about love of self and maintaining a balance in your life so you can go the distance with the least amount of harm.

Differentiation is the first step in moving towards a person having the ability to self-soothe, self-regulate and self-direct, which is discussed further in Chapter 16.

Control

Control, or having 'controlling behaviour', is a description that can be damaging to a person in a family that perceives themselves as really trying to do the right thing. A professor of clinical psychology, Dr L. Parrott, describes the basic issue that underlies control as anxiety.[5] His research findings were that the motivations or dynamics underlying the need to control are fuelled by the anxiety that runs the engine of control. This anxiety translates into fear. For carers, anxiety or fear can be caused or driven by concerns about their competency to care, their fear of the future, feeling unsupported, legal and financial issues in the family, criticism about how they care, the uncertainty of the length of time that they will be required to care, whether or not their care is good enough, and their physical health.

When I hear a person being described as 'controlling' or 'a control freak' I begin to look for possible causes of anxiety or fears that could be underpinning the need to control the behaviour of the person with dementia. Once the fears have been explored and listed you can move on to the next level and address other issues such as trust, meaning trust in letting go of some of the aspects of care and then being able to delegate some of the responsibility of caring. When you are caught in the slipstream of caring it is difficult to step back and take an objective view or become aware of just what it is that drives your anxiety and hence your need to control. Control of others is a defensive mechanism that keeps you safe on one hand and caged in the other. Sometimes it feels like there is no solution, but don't worry—there always is.

13 Attachment and non-attachment

AS PART OF THE HUMAN RACE WE NEED TO BE ATTACHED TO someone or something to make sense of our world. You only have to turn on the television or visit someone in their home to see photographs depicting attachments: the couple, the graduate, the new mother and baby, the family reunion, the school photograph, Fido the much loved dog or a basket of kittens. People carry symbolic attachments to the workplace—photographs sit on desks and garage walls. Attachments are part of your identity and they remind you of who you are, where you came from and where you would like to go as well as what you value.

When does attachment begin?

Children attach to their mothers for survival. At birth their mother is their world—she stands for the continued existence of the child. The mother feeds, holds, smells and smiles and has the capacity to give and to take away, to soothe and frustrate.

Animals know which is their offspring: ewes can find their lamb in a nursery, a foal can find its mother in the paddock, a bird will throw an interloper out of the nest. This programming of nature has propagated the world, and will continue to do so. Consider this much quoted saying: 'There is no such thing as a baby—only a mother and a baby together.'[1]

Children with a secure attachment to their mother tend to grow up and form similar secure attachments. This forms the basis of an adult being able to develop a strong sense of self. The less fortunate child who has an unavailable parent may be so concerned with staying close to the parent that they are unable to play and therefore find their inner self, leading to difficulties with attachments. The child's sense of self can become compromised, always doing or thinking what should be done rather than what they need to do for themselves.

In the process of growing up, the child can form attachments to other members in the family, to society, community, the state and the nation. Attachment is not something that we grow out of when we reach adulthood. When faced with anxiety or fear, people will automatically seek out other people to support them the same way a child does when separated from its mother. The child searches for reassurance, and once found moves on to play happily.

Individual and family attachments

A psychosocial assessment is useful in identifying family attachments. Families vary greatly, in size, personal strengths, health, beliefs about care and commitment to caring. One way to identify unique family diversity is to interview family members either as a group or individually. Family therapists who use a Bowenian systems approach routinely use a genogram, an intergenerational family tree or map (see page 165) that is helpful in recognising family characteristics and opens up a lot of information. Family members do not always recognise that other life issues have an impact on the person with dementia and the carer. For example, if there has been an untimely death such as a suicide or an accident, or there is a person with a disability, family conflict, drug and alcohol problems, an unplanned retirement or financial problems. These real life issues would have been impacting on the family prior to the diagnosis; after the diagnosis, the family becomes more stressed.

The genogram not only shows who is related to whom in the way of a family tree, but more importantly how they relate to each other. Who loves or hates whom, or is indifferent, or which family member may have been cut off from the family for many years.

Patterns of attachments between family members soon become quite clear, as do family members that are not attached or are attached by varying degrees. Behind each strong attachment there will often be a story of how and why this occurred. How or why people take on the role of care or their level of commitment to care has consequences for how well the caregiver can adjust to the task of caring and still remain mentally and physically healthy.

Other social issues that need to be included in the family assessment include changes to the financial situation, legal matters, role changes, occupational or housing choices. Each family will have their own issues, but these decisions will be affected by how attached the caregiver is to the person with the dementing illness; that is, they can be overinvolved or overattached and forget that they will have their own needs and may not be able to sustain as high a level of care as was at first thought possible. This commonly results in feelings of guilt and personal incompetence.

The carer comes first

There are many levels and a variety of strategies required to adapt to new situations that occur when there is a person with dementia in the family. The situation can be helped if you begin by putting yourself first. Although this doesn't sound right, the best thing you can do is to be informed, and to be physically and mentally in good shape. This idea flies in the face of all prior learning about care. The self-depre-cating model of people standing around a bed, powerless, waiting for instructions from the good doctor or fading away to a shadow of their former selves is a negative image of care in this century. The over-responsible carer refuses to go out of the house because something might happen to the person with dementia. Is this productive?

Understanding some of the basics of attachment theory can make sense of the need to move from the outer world of the caregiver to the inner world of the self, into one's distinctive and unique inner world. It is from this point that a person can regain or begin to develop a sense of entitlement, not to the disadvantage of others but from a mature sense of who we are and of our own worth. This leads to the capacity for achieving both intimacy with others and mastery of ourselves.

Fear and anxiety

All adults experience many fears and anxieties. The environment and social order have changed more in the last thirty years than in the previous 300 years.[2] The change of pace and technology and the lack of a consistent set of standards and values leaves a vacuum in which people are left to fend for themselves. The daily diet of media infor-mation that pours forth twenty-four hours a day lacks any context or a view of the wider picture. A two-minute coverage of a disaster that kills fifty innocent victims is followed by an advertisement for run-ning shoes, drinking chocolate or a seven-day holiday at a bargain price. Where does all this information go? It has been suggested that anxiety disorders (being the number one mental health problem among women) are simply the outcome of a diminished ability to cope with the stress and fears of modern daily life.

Common fears expressed by carers following the diagnosis of a dementing illness include:

- fear of separation;
- sadness about loss;
- anger and protest about separation;
- rage and guilt in response to trauma;
- jealousy of people who seem to be closer to the person of importance to us;
- fear of losing the person, as they had previously known them;
- fear of the unknown;
- fear of the future;
- fear of the stigma of dementia;
- fear of being isolated; and
- fear of the person with dementia being forgotten by friends and family.

This list of fears is an indication of some of the concerns that people express. These fears can immobilise the carer of a family. One young wife reported that:

> *It has taken me six months to even begin to comprehend what I am supposed to be doing or even consider the future responsibilities.*

I am always bemused by the catchphrase 'get a life'. If you don't understand why you can't or don't get a life then it is stupidity in its highest form. Getting a life is a process of learning how to detach while still attached or connected (in this case) to the person with dementia.

Attachment is a theory that sees the individual not in isolation but in a relationship. First with their primary relationship, then to others in the family such as the father, siblings, grandparents, uncles, aunts and cousins, then to a wider society. Each circle offers both security and insecurity.

If a person has pre-existing physical, personal, relationship or social problems such as unemployment or illness in the family, then these issues over time create feelings of insecurity. Feelings of insecurity are often not understood, but can be expressed in certain behaviours such as doing things to excess, eating, sleeping, shopping, incurring debts, working, unsafe driving and the overuse of alcohol and drugs for physical ailments such as headaches, stiff necks, backaches or skin conditions. Many people seek treatment for their ailments but rarely stop to reflect upon the cause and possible remedy.

Understanding the concept of attachment can help you make sense of the significance of losses or potential losses in your life.

Good attachment in the early years is extremely important as it gives you nurturing and freedom from anxiety so you can move on to a higher order of being in the world. The need for secure attachment to something or someone continues your whole life be it a place, a belief, a god, a person or an animal—something that you can reach out to for solace, meaning, purpose and comfort. The secret is to find the balance between attachment and non-attachment, two sides of the one coin.

Non-attachment and detachment for the caregiver

People often think that being non-attached means not caring or not loving. The opposite feeling to love is indifference—which is very, very different to being non-attached. Non-attachment has been described as the ability to be non-possessive, not ambivalent, autonomous, freely entering into attachment, in which the object is held and cherished but not controlled.[3] This non-attachment is based upon respect and choice, rather than where you have attachment based upon fear and anxiety about the present and future. Non-attachment allows you to focus on the moment, to pay attention to the now.

Having the ability to still your fears, or having an inner peace of detachment, creates a sense of self that disallows external happenings to influence your behaviour. This is not about not caring for others; rather, it is a way to obtain clarity about yourself, and thus wisdom. This sense of your autonomy goes hand in hand with appropriate boundaries between self and others. Maintaining an inner and outer balance is a lifelong challenge. Most religions of the world recommend the daily practice of prayer, meditation or daily reflection to assist people to re-establish or reconnect with their centre or spirit and to see themselves as an important cog in a much larger wheel.

Attachment and the person with dementia

Around the time of diagnosis and beyond, people with dementia are often depressed or behave in different ways. Depression can in part cause behavioural changes, however, with the gradual loss of cognitive ability that dementia causes it is most likely that they will be acutely experiencing a loss of what was safe or familiar in their environment. Looking at the face of a person that they have known for years and not being able to remember their name is one such instance.

This experience of being in an insecure and frightening world activates similar patterns of behaviour to the attachment behaviours seen in very young children when they encounter a new situation.[4] Children will check out Mum and Dad's face for reassurance when they are in a new situation. Likewise for the person with dementia when unsure or fearful. Having to confront fears of the unknown many times in a single day will in time lead to behavioural changes in the person with dementia, such as 'shadowing' or not wanting the carer to leave them, or repetitive questions about arrangements, dates and times for things. Once the cause of the anxiety is understood, an appropriate response to the person with dementia is more readily adjusted to. The paradox of this situation is that the carer is revisiting attachment issues of their own such as fear of being left alone, loss of the person as they knew them, and the loss of a planned future. The person with dementia often shows their anxiety and fear in behavioural ways, especially in the early stages when they may have lost the ability to express themselves verbally as well as they did in the past.

14 Counselling

MANY PEOPLE BELIEVE THAT COUNSELLING CAN BE ACHIEVED BY filling out a questionnaire in a magazine. Others may believe that it is a risky business baring your soul to a total stranger. And why should you? Because something in your life is hurting and affecting your peace of mind and inevitably those people around you. Counselling gives you the opportunity to have a confidential conversation with a person who is unbiased because they do not have any investment in the outcome. They will not discuss your personal issues with other people and they have the training and ability to shed a different light on the situation. Having a professional person to walk with you as you make life choices is both comforting and reassuring.

People often get concerned over the difference between therapy and counselling. Counselling involves a one-to-one relationship between the counsellor and the person seeking help, whereas therapy is the process that is used in counselling to unlock the secret causes of a person's discomfort that are often not consciously available or have been forgotten over time.

Effective counselling offers people another way of looking at a problem, or it offers another story within which they can make sense of their difficulties. That, in itself, produces an enhanced sense of mastery and control over their situation. Put another way, if life events create a disconnection from a person's sense of self-worth, self-control and mastery, counselling is a process that assists people to reconnect with their hidden strengths and inherent wisdom.

People don't have difficulties solving their own situations because they are not clever or wise. It is more likely that they are too close to the wood to be able to see the trees. Often issues are just too confronting. Another tricky issue is that much of how you feel and what you do or think comes from your unconscious, that part of your brain that you cannot readily access without a skilled therapist. People have been reared to think logically or sequentially that if 'this' happens it is because of 'that'. That may be so on the surface, but if the problem persists it may be fuelled by unconscious material. Family beliefs that are not useful in this unique situation with dementia usually cause the sticking point that hinders progress.

One of the tenets of systemic therapy is to maintain a healthy curiosity; a healthy curiosity means that therapists:

- Never assume that they understand anything.
- Need to explore what meaning this 'event' has for the client.
- Will thoroughly unpack the layers of meaning.
- Will constantly maintain a therapeutic stance that allows them to remain focused on the client's story but unattached to the problem.
- Identify the dominant and recurring themes in the client's story as a basis for therapy and change.
- Will reframe the presenting problem in such a way that it invites the client to think about it from a different perspective.
- Will acknowledge the positive attempts to change the situation that people have been doing prior to coming for counselling.

The therapy actually happens in the course of the person's daily life, as ideas discussed in the formal session become fertile soil for new perceptions and understandings, thus enabling attitudinal and behavioural changes.

The following case histories give a snapshot of what can occur during a counselling session. These case histories are not real, but they have been compiled from many case histories of many families that have the same theme occurring.

Case history 1: Bag's been packed for years

Bill, aged sixty-three, was referred by his local doctor for a counselling appointment when he found out that his 58-year-old wife Cynthia was diagnosed with Alzheimer's disease. Bill described their communication as having been non-existent for the past four years, and their sexual relationship as being 'dead in the water' for the last ten years. He had been planning to leave Cynthia when he retired and take a caravan and disappear. He enjoyed his job as a steel worker and as he was away from home for ten to twelve hours per day he could for the most part ignore the domestic situation. He played squash three times a week, and saw himself as fit and healthy. He took separate holidays and visited his only son in America once a year for about three weeks. He felt close to his son, but over the years they had made a pact not to discuss Cynthia. 'He knows how it is, so there is no use going over old ground.' There was no third party involved.

Possible themes that the therapist could explore include loyalty, commitment, ambivalence, anger, resentment, the financial implications, love, hope, the possibility of a reconciliation, safe routine, non-risk, indifference, unresolved conflictual relationship patterns, and the family of origin patterns of communication.

In the first session we looked at the time around the diagnosis, and how it had occurred. Cynthia had a girlfriend that she spent a lot of time with; the friend had mentioned to Bill that Cynthia was having problems with her memory and she was concerned about her.

Bill had advised the friend to do what she could and left it at that. The friend had accompanied Cynthia to the doctor and then to see a neuropsychologist for tests. She told Bill what was happening over the ensuing months while the testing continued and then, finally, Bill was asked to come and see the doctor with Cynthia.

The doctor told them that Cynthia was in the early stages of dementia, and it would be a good idea if they contacted the Alzheimer's Association for support and counselling. He would be available if were there any problems, but he would like to see Cynthia in three months. Cynthia commenced anti-depressant medication, as the doctor was of the opinion that she was clinically depressed. They left the surgery together and when they arrived home Cynthia had phoned her friend and then her son. They had not had any further discussion about the diagnosis since then. The following questions were put to Bill.

What attracted you to her in the first place. Where did you meet?
We met on an apple farm, picking in the fruit season. She was waiting to go into nursing, and I was waiting to hear if I had a job at an iron foundry. We had both gone fruit picking just for fun. One night they held a barbecue for all the pickers and I asked her to dance. She was a country girl and I was from the city. We became engaged quite quickly and married about three years later.

What was it like in the beginning of your marriage?
Good. We were both hard workers, good savers, and I built our home back in the early 1960s.

Did you have any family nearby?
No, they all lived abroad—we visited them each year for Christmas, especially after our son Arthur was born. They all wanted to see him.

What about Cynthia's family? Where were they living?
On the farm, they were country people and rarely if ever came to town.

How did you keep in contact with them?
Cynthia did all that kind of thing, until her parents were killed in a car accident about ten years after we were married. Her elder brother Ben and his family took over the farm and things started to go downhill from there.

Downhill in what way?
I am not sure. I was never close to Ben, but from where I stood it seemed that Cynthia was doing all the contacting and then it fizzled out. We became Darby and Joan. We just puddled along.

It must have been awful for her, losing all her family—how did she cope?
I am not sure really.

Did she look to you for support?
Yes, well I went to the funeral, and I put up the money for the headstones and that sort of thing. Yes, I did support her.

Did she have any other family to support her?
No.

Friends?
Yes. There was always Joan, her friend from school who lives just around the corner. She looked after her, she was always at home so I guess they sorted it out between them.

Did you ever feel left out?
No, not really. I felt sorry for her but I knew that I could not fix things. I worked and supplied the money for her to do whatever she wanted to. She did not have any financial worries, or things like that.

At this point in the session I would introduce the idea of drawing a family tree of three to four generations so I could get an idea about the family patterns and history. The presenting problem can then be explored in a wider family context.

Bill had one brother, who had been killed at the age of eighteen in a motorbike accident. His parents were still alive, but kept to themselves. His father had been a plumber and had retired at the age of seventy and now occupied himself with racing pigeons. His mother was involved in the church and they rarely left the small town where they had lived for most of their lives. His father was the eldest of five children but, following the death of his parents, the boys had not kept in contact with each other and saw one another only at Christmas and funerals.

He described his uncles as hard-working men who were good providers but were emotionally quite distant from each other. They were the strong silent types.

What do you imagine sustained them? What was the light that kept them going?
I am not sure. They never appeared to need anybody. They just kept themselves to themselves.

Was your father like that?
Most likely. He never appeared to have any needs at all come to think of it.

When your parents fought, who won?
My dad would yell and dance around for a while, and then all would be quiet and then things went back to normal.

How did your father show that he cared for your mother?
I am not sure. She never wanted for anything though. She always said that there was enough money in the bank for her to run away around the world if she wanted to.

What do you think stopped her from doing just that?
She may have thought that Dad would turn into a pigeon and fly away while she was gone! (Laughs.)

So if your mum left for a holiday she was worried that when she came back your dad may have flown the coop, so to speak.
Yes.

So while your mum had the money she was also stuck because of her fear that he would not be there for her when she returned?
Yes. When he went to the war she said that she never wanted to go through that time of not knowing ever again in her life. It was like living with your heart in your mouth for three years. It left her a changed woman.

Counselling objectives

The objectives when counselling Bill would be to:

- Gain an understanding of what had kept Bill in the marriage, and what had stopped him from leaving his wife many years ago.
- Find out what he wanted to do now. Did he want assistance to leave, or be supported to stay and care for his wife?
- Demonstrate to Bill how his family patterns of disengagement and isolation or emotional shutdown towards significant others was not new. He had been surrounded by it all his life.
- Indicate that as children one of the many tasks we have is to gain a sense of self. If that is not successfully achieved then in later life we will unconsciously choose a partner with whom the early inter-action between self and mother will be re-created and re-experienced. If Bill's mother was concerned about being on her own it is highly likely that Bill may have some of the same uncon-scious fears.
- Instil hope for himself and a sense of how well he has fulfilled his objective in being a good provider.

The relationship problems in this marriage could have gone on for many years except that the diagnosis of dementia has created a catalyst. We would further explore the implication of staying and like-wise the implications of going. If Bill chooses to stay he will not be able to stay as a self-sufficient 'island' but will be required to partici-pate in a much more meaningful way.

Bill left this session to think about his decision. If he chooses to stay I would like to see them both as a couple, in the hope that some change can occur and part of the young girl and young man that met in the orchard can be rekindled.

Doing couple therapy when one of the partners has been diag-nosed with dementia, requires the therapist to slow the pace down and give each person equal time to speak. The therapist should ask other oriented questions: such as how Cynthia thinks Bill feels about the changes in her behaviour like her frustration over memory loss and whether or not Bill sees her behaviour in the same way.

Other oriented questions are asked to clarify the perception that each person has of the problem. It allows both parties to hear the differences or similarities about a situation that could be a cause of a marital conflict, as often people believe that they both think the same.

Couple counselling objectives

The objectives when couselling Bill and Cynthia as a couple would be to:

- Develop an understanding of the impact of the dementia on the couple's relationship.
- Determine adjustments needed to be made to accommodate changes caused by the disease.
- Clarify each other's perspectives.
- Validate each other's feeling.
- Normalise their experiences.
- Acknowledge differences.

The light that once shone between this couple has diminished over the years to a tiny flicker that splutters like an indecisive candle. The list of hurts or wrongdoings, disappointments and the loss of dreams sits in their chest like a stone in the bottom of the pool. They are unhappy, miserable—and stuck.

If their relationship problem can be reframed in a different light, they may choose to stay together after the cards have been placed on the table and assessed individually. Even if this couple dissolve the relationship it will be with the knowledge that they have looked at both the similarities and the differences.

Case history 2: Is it love or is it the inheritance?

Older people with early stage dementia can often continue to live and function quite well on their own with minimal support from their family, until something happens such as a sudden illness or an accident. Hospitalisation or an anaesthetic can be the time when a previously coping elder person appears to have changed overnight. The change of environment and the drugs used for anaesthetic along with the shock of the injury can result in disorientation and confusion for varying lengths of time.

A family huddle frequently occurs and a family member will be chosen or will volunteer to move in with the parent for rehabilitation purposes. This is most likely to be the child with the least amount of family commitments.

Mrs P, aged seventy-four, had lived alone for the past eight years after the death of her husband. She had been a socially active person involved in community groups and the church and regularly took bus trips to points of interest. Over the past two years she had dropped many of her activities, saying that she was past it and now was only attending her local church each Sunday and the ladies' guild meeting once a month. She still did her own shopping and housework.

After an accident, it was decided (by the family) that Sybil, her middle daughter, who was divorced, would move in to take care of her until she was back on her feet. Time passed and the rehabilitation progressed uneventfully but slowly. Sybil discovered some strange things in the home that she described as downright dangerous, like twenty containers of bleach under the sink in unmarked containers, plastic bags by the hundreds stored in a back bedroom, and food stashed in the laundry cupboard that would last her mother for years. Sybil gave up her full-time job as a primary school teacher as her mother required full-time care.

For some unknown reason Sybil took it upon herself to have her mother agree to give her sole power of attorney without discussing this step with her other two siblings, Susan and Jane. At a family dinner some six months later, Susan, the youngest daughter, suggested that getting a power of attorney over her mother's (substantial) financial affairs might be a provident step. Sybil told her that a power of attorney had already been taken care of as she had discovered that their mother had been taking large sums of money out of the bank two or three times a week and that she was angry with the bank for not telling someone in the family about their mother's behaviour, so she had taken her mother to her solicitor and arranged an enduring power of attorney.

The other sisters understood the problem with their mother's memory but were puzzled by the one-sided decision taken by their sister. Sybil's view was that when their mother needed a carer it automatically included all aspects of her mother's life, not just being the taxi service, chief cook and bottle washer. Sybil said:

> *Being a carer is a full-time job, you can't just walk out the door when you feel like it, you don't always have a night's uninterrupted sleep. I spend my life going from one appointment with Mother to the next. This is not a complaint—it is reality. How do you imagine I was going to run around to see all of you each*

time a cheque needed to be drawn to pay a household account?
The house does not run itself. I have given up my work to take
over this role when no one else put up his or her hand for the
job. In fact, who else has actually been to see Mother on a reg-
ular basis? It's only now that you have decided that Mother's
financial affairs need attention that what I do or have done has
your attention.

Needless to say the convivial dinner ground to an abrupt halt
as the information percolated through the brains of the other family
members.

The following day the second daughter phoned Sybil to say that
the other members of the family wanted to meet and discuss her decision to take out power of attorney in her own name without consulting
any of them. Sybil declined the offer to meet as she was too busy at
the present time but would let them know later when she would be
available.

The family cohesion now had a fracture: was it care and concern
versus power and control?

Possible themes that the therapist could explore include trust,
ambivalence, retribution, power and control versus care and control,
grief—anticipated loss of the mother, loss of marriage, unresolved
family conflict, secrets, middle child syndrome, ambiguous loss, shame,
conflicting beliefs and values about care and long-standing communication problems.

Each case history presents the therapist with interpretations of
the events that have created the problem in the family. In order for
a change or shift to occur the therapist keeps a stance of curiosity
about some of the possible themes that need to be explored in each
session.

Everyone creates their own reality of a problem by looking at a
situation from their point of view. This viewpoint may not contain
all the facts and therefore over time become skewed. The longer the

problem exists, the greater the likelihood that you become even more attached to your 'truth'.

This family had reached a stalemate; once this state is reached, usually one of the family members will phone the Alzheimer's Association and seek information about the mother's dementia and how it could progress. At the first session the above-mentioned scenario gets tabled.

Families are complex entities and 'how they cope may be dysfunctional, but it is not the same as saying that the person or the family is dysfunctional'.[1] In the absence of clarity people will take whatever action they deem necessary to keep things on an even keel. In this situation Sybil took action—so she could manage her mother's financial affairs and not bother the family. You could take the hypothetical view that Sybil was experiencing ambiguous loss and one way that she could have some control over the situation was by taking out enduring power of attorney to ensure that her mother was not being ripped off by greedy people.

Counselling objectives

The objectives when counselling this family would be to:

- Provide each member of the family with a safe, non-judgmental place to express their concerns about the problem.
- Clarify Sybil's behaviour, which seemed so out of character.
- Explore how trust as a virtue has been tested in the family prior to this event.
- Ascertain why they had sought help for this problem now and not sooner.
- Explore the family's covert or overt beliefs about caring for a parent.
- Find out which daughter was the most affected by the mother's diagnosis of dementia and why.
- Discover if there were any 'rules' about care, or were there any offers of respite for Sybil to help her to reconstruct her life following her divorce.

- Find out if intimacy was expressed in the family.

Counselling objectives are not static, but change continuously. Having a list of questions to guide an interview keeps the therapist as neutral as possible as new information comes to light that has previously not been considered.

Susan and Jane attended the first counselling session. Both told their story from their perspective, and what emerged was the unanimous disappointment at Sybil for taking matters into her own hand. The two sisters sided together against the middle sister. They acknowledged that she had been doing an excellent job as carer but, had they known of her decision, they would have paid closer attention to the situation and not let this get out of hand.

At the end of the session I told them how impressed I was that they had chosen to seek a solution to the problem, as it takes courage to seek solutions rather than see the problem from one view. I wondered if Sybil had taken this action as a way of gaining some control over a situation with which she was possibly feeling out of control?

In the second session I was curious to find out how their mother having a dementing illness was affecting them individually. Jane said that it was dreadful but that they would manage, as they had coped with their father's cancer and had nursed him at home until he had died. The questioning continued.

How was that different to what is happening to you now?
I guess we felt that what we did was appreciated, but with Mother it is as if she does not care if we are there or not.

And when this happens how does this affect you?
Jane: I feel that being with her is a waste of time really. I can't get through to her like Sybil can.

What does Sybil do that is different?

I don't know. She seems to have an uncanny way of understanding what Mum needs, and they laugh a lot.

About what?

I don't know—silly things. Like Mum hid the car keys in the fridge and Sybil thought that it was funny. Or one day Mum locked herself in the toilet, and after calling a handyman Sybil made camp outside the bathroom door and sang songs to Mum until she was released. Mum follows Sybil around a lot of the time and Sybil thinks that's okay. She takes Mum to the heated pool for physiotherapy twice a week, and I really don't understand why she bothers. I can't see how it helps, but Sybil thinks it is good for both of them. Sybil wants to keep fit, and she thinks Mum should be fit also. They dance along to the music—sometimes I wonder who has the dementia.

So you don't agree with Sybil's recipe for care?

Parts of it are okay, but sometimes I don't agree with what she does. But then I am not in her position. She has always had the capacity to see the funny side of things.

Where do you imagine that Sybil gets her wisdom for being able to cope with your mum's changed behaviour from?

Perhaps because she is a teacher.

Do they teach dementia care at university?

No, but kids do similar things.

Like what?

They follow you around, they forget things or leave them in strange places.

How do you imagine that Sybil copes with seeing your mum get distressed when her memory fails her?
I don't know.

Have you ever asked her?
No.

How come?
I can't cope with it myself, let alone ask her what it is like for her.

What part of your mum's dementia do you have difficulty coping with?
Most of it really. I just see the end—her not knowing me.

That must be really difficult for you—feeling that you can't share with your sister the loss of your mother as you had known her.
(Silence, followed by tears.) I am sorry about this.

It's okay, just take your time.
(Silence for a few minutes.)

I am so impressed that you have chosen to share your sadness with me today, it must be so difficult for you to have hung on to your sadness for so long. Perhaps one day you might share how you feel with your sister. My hunch is that she is feeling as isolated as you are and her taking out enduring power of attorney was a feature of how isolated and lonely she has been feeling.

Susan, Sybil, and Jane all attended the third session. There was a relaxed feeling in the room and Sybil was welcomed to the session.

Jane: Well, you opened up a can of worms after the last session. Sue and I left here and went for coffee and talked for hours. We decided that we would not invite Sybil to another meeting—we would go to her without our families. We realised that this was our mother and we needed to understand what Sybil was doing and why.

Sybil: This pair arrived and said they wanted to have a chat with Mum present. They apologised for their lack of support and attention, and said that they were actually scared as they did not know just what to do, or how to do it. I was stunned. Mum did not grasp it all but she appeared to get the message about how they felt, she smiled and gave them a big hug. We all started to cry. It was amazing. It was the best thing that has happened to us since the diagnosis. I felt that we were connected again as we had been in the past. I told them about my divorce and how I had felt such a failure and that my self-esteem was so low. Becoming Mum's carer served a few altruistic purposes. I felt that it was something that I could make a success of. I had the time and the desire to do a good job. However, after I took on the job I felt that I was being left to do all of the work, without any recognition from them. A weekly phone call is really not enough. I thought, she is your mother too and where are you now?

Sybil's disclosure of her position and her fears were explored further and it was agreed that each child would take turns in the care of their mother, offering Sybil time out on a regular basis. They left the session with the intention of going home to make up a calendar showing their mother's appointments and recreational activities (including the heated pool) and work out a way that they could all contribute to the best of their capabilities.

Trust and cohesion had begun to be restored. It had never actually been lost, just put on hold as they turned another corner in life. These women were searching for solutions to what had happened to their relationships. People who have good intentions and want solutions are very likely to find them.

Family hurts can run silently and deeply for a long time, until some event provides an opening for a change. Sybil's legal action gained a response from her sisters that could have led to an ongoing family feud over the potential loss of the inheritance or loss of financial control. The intervention used here is called a reframe, which is a therapeutic technique that enables clients to see the meaning of their situation differently. The setting or viewpoint of a situation is placed 'in another frame which fits the "facts" of the same concrete situation equally well or even better, and thereby changes its entire meaning'.[2]

Seeking professional outside help can achieve positive results as the family actually has many strengths that may have been temporarily forgotten under the weight of commitments, work, child care and fear of the unknown. Focusing on the obvious injustice only furthers and deepens the problem, as it is common practice to take a lineal view of the problem and react to a one-dimensional view. Having the courage to address your own fears allows you to begin understanding some of the rationale behind other people's behaviour. This is the key element in creating opportunities for a cooperative and collaborative care.

Providing a safe place for people to express their fears and sense of loss is the first step towards finding solutions to family dilemmas.

Case history 3: The only child

Only children have a unique position when they become carers for a dementing parent. Some have families of their own, others don't. Some are still rearing children and some are in the position or family life cycle where they are looking forward to finding a life for themselves, or perhaps looking forward to having time for themselves to pursue a long awaited hobby.

Julie, aged forty-two, requested a counselling session to find out how she could cope with her parents. Her 68-year-old father was a retired optometrist and was very involved in stamp collecting and golf. His 65-year-old wife had recently been diagnosed with vascular dementia following many years of having hypertension. Julie's concern was that the house was a mess and her father refused to have any outside help.

She described him as being spoilt by her mother and his mother prior to their marriage forty-three years ago. When she visited her parents each weekend she saw that the tasks that her mother had always done such as cleaning out the fridge and the top of the stove were no longer being done. Her father was happy for her to do the cleaning but was extremely reluctant to have outsider help.

Julie worked as a doctor's receptionist and often had to refer patients to community services, so she was familiar with what was available in her parents' community. Her father, however, could not see that there was a problem (inferring that Julie could clean the house on weekends when she came to visit) and refused all services.

Julie's long-term relationship had broken up the year prior and she was slowly coming to terms with the loss. She had joined the local tennis club and played each Saturday afternoon. She needed to work full-time to support herself.

Julie understood that eventually she would be the most likely person to care for her parents, but at the moment she was not prepared to become the full-time housekeeper because her father could. However, he refused to take on the domestic role that was now required.

Julie described her relationship with her mother prior to the diagnosis as being all right. She had always disagreed with the way her mother was possessive of her father and treated him like some kind of demigod. Her mother had had periods of depression over the last few years and said that she was worried about the fact that Julie was not married and would have no one to look after her.

Her mother had begun to exhibit some personality changes and had become abusive and overly emotional. In response to her mother's change of behaviour her father became more engrossed in his hobbies and distanced himself from her. Julie felt like the meat in the sandwich.

Possible themes that a therapist could explore include anger, depression, denial, guilt, powerlessness, power and control, ambivalence, lack of knowledge about what dementia means to her father, adjustments— coping with personality changes and the emotional and verbal abuse, the systemic pattern—a sequence of interactions of a couple or family that becomes repetitive over time,[3] loss of personal space and time, the divided loyalties or differentiation of self, the family role and role reversal, ambiguous loss, core beliefs about caring—how much is enough, and gender issues—is caring best done by females?

One other issue is triangulation, the process whereby any two-party relationship which is experiencing great intensity will naturally involve a third party to reduce anxiety. This can be a person, issue, substance or any entity that takes the focus off the relationship and thereby reduces the tension.[4]

Theoretical models: Systemic and solution-focused brief therapy

The therapist could ask Julie to list which of her concerns she rated as the most pressing or the most problematical for her at present. She could then be asked if there were any significant other people around the family that she could enlist for support. There could also be exploration around how the diagnosis occurred, and what role was played during the diagnostic process would be pursued.

Counselling objectives

The objectives when counselling Julie would be to:

- Gain an understanding of the relationship between her parents.

- Find out what role Julie wanted to have with her mother's care.

- Reframe the presenting problem for Julie to see her father's indifference as fear.

- Understand the possible reasons that her father was reluctant to receive outside assistance with housecleaning.

- Understand and, if appropriate, validate her feeling about being the meat in the sandwich.

- Normalise the role that only children are often conscripted into when one parent has dementia and there are no other family members to contribute to the caring.

- Explore further Julie's thoughts about her mother's depression and beliefs that if Julie was married she would be taken care of given her mother's situation.

- Support Julie through her own issues about the pending loss of a parent.

- Explain behavioural and personality changes that can occur in the early, middle and later stages of dementia.

- Ascertain if Julie's parents would join her in a counselling session.

At the first session Julie said that she had been the first person to notice her mother's forgetfulness and said that she thought that it was due to her being depressed. After a few months, when her mother did not appear to be getting any better, she mentioned her concerns to her father. He said that she was suffering from 'imaginitis'. Julie pursued and finally achieved a referral to a geriatrician. Julie said she had to ask her father about the results from the MRI scan and he had reluctantly told her the diagnosis was early stage dementia.

Following re-engagement with Julie, the second session was linked back to the time of her mother's diagnosis. These questions were asked.

What happened then?

Mum was very upset and wondered who was going to look after Dad. I said that he would be fine and for her not to worry. She seemed happy with that. But later she asked me again, 'What about Dad?' I again told her that he would be fine. I felt awful at that stage because I really had no idea how he would cope, but I just trusted that when the time came we would muddle through things together.

Did you speak with your father about how he felt?
I tried to and he said that it was not a big deal at the moment and to leave it alone.

Is that how he usually manages problems?
This is the first problem that he has had, at home that is.

What did you do after your dad gave his opinion?
I went home and thought, maybe he is right. What could I do? But then I thought, well, she is my mum and when she needs care I can get some help for Dad.

What do you imagine is getting in the way of your father accepting some outside help?
He is just stubborn and spoilt.

What do you think about the idea that his denial or his lack of insight has a functional purpose in that he may be frightened and overwhelmed by the thought of losing his wife as he knows her and of what the future may hold for him. What if we saw his denial as taking some time out until he can begin to come to terms with her diagnosis. At the moment he can stay with his denial if he can conscript you into taking over where your mother has left off, but if it continues it could be harmful to his mental health. It has the downside of leaving your dad isolated from reality and stops other people supporting him in an adult way. He will lose his power by needing to manipulate you into doing things that he could either do for himself or pay for some other person to do. Sometimes it is difficult for children to see their parents needing assistance but refusing to accept any help outside of themselves.
Yes, I feel that I could be dragged in to do everything and he would just let me do it all. I feel so angry that he wants me as an adult to do the housework, and be a child when it suits him.

Can you tell me how your parents sorted out the marital problems that occur from time to time in most relationships?
Oh! Yes. Mum would phone me and say that Dad did xyz and she was so mad with him!

And what did you do then?
It depended on the situation. Sometimes I would phone Dad and tell him how Mum felt.

And what happened then?
Dad usually apologised to Mum and everything was sweet.

How did you find out that things were back to normal?
Mum would tell me.

What do you imagine would have happened if you had not become your mum's advocate?
Oh! I don't know—I have always done it. I guess they would have sorted it out somewhere along the track.

Can you see any similarities between the problem that you are having now and what used to happen in the past?
Yes, I guess that I am having a problem with Dad and Mum can't advocate for me. The tables have turned. I now understand how she must have felt, and why she phoned me all the time.

What else do you think your mum could have done rather than phone you when she was having problems with your dad?
She could have spoken up for herself.

What stopped her from doing that do you think?
She knew I could get through to Dad more easily than she could.

Why was that?
Because he loved me and did not want me to be upset.

Right. So you have held the solutions to your parent's problems for many years now?
I guess so.

So having your dad turn to you for support would be about normal for him in the bigger scheme of things?
Yes, but I am not prepared to give up my life for his needs right now. I will care and support them both, but I am entitled to a life.

I had been waiting for that strong woman to stand up, and here she was. This is good, but it is not a long-term solution because the behavioural patterns between Julie and her parents have been firmly established for many years. Change needs to be taken gently. I asked Julie what she thought about negotiating with her father just like she had always done in the past.

I told Julie to tell her father how concerned she was about her mother and that she really wanted to be around to help him now and in the years to come. If he was prepared to have someone come in to clean the house each fortnight, Julie would be free to take her mother out each Saturday morning (if convenient for Julie) so he could go and do his own thing. So Julie could have quality time with her mum, and her dad could either go along or take time out. This would serve the dual purpose of letting him know that she would be around, and would let him know that she understood that it is not always easy for him to ask for his needs to be met. If he has always had someone else to smooth things over it is unhelpful to apportion blame. He will in time regain his confidence and self-esteem but it the meantime a strategic approach can save face as well as free up the lines of communication that are the basis of good relationships.

15 Looking after yourself

THE CENTRAL THEMES OF THIS BOOK ARE ABOUT THE BRAIN, early intervention and an equal partnership between the person with a dementing illness and their carer. The brain of the person that you care for is of equal importance to yours. As a carer, over time, you will become the substitute memory for the person with dementia. You may be coping with repetitive questions, repetitive actions and heightened distractibility. This will take up your mental energy and you will be thinking for two people, just as you did if you had a child.

This chapter explores some ways that may assist you to keep your mind in good working condition. If you have not paid any particular attention to your mental fitness, now is the time to seriously consider getting it into as good a shape as possible. A carer's proactive thinking is a healthier outcome than reactive behaviour, which signals that one is out of control. You cannot give what you do not have.

Architects create plans for builders to follow so they will end up with something similar to what the customer had in mind. Caring is not so different: all the life issues that will be affected following the diagnosis could be considered in a logical step-by-step process. This does not involve looking too far ahead, but rather having a manageable plan that provides time to think about situations, to discuss issues with other people and to find out about services and their costs. Doing these things provides one way of moving from a situation that seems overwhelming to one where you can consider specific questions in a more concrete way. This process will need to be reviewed as events change. It is important to share your findings with the family— if you have one, if they will listen, and if you have a relationship with them.

A mental health care plan

Caring for a person with dementia requires a plan that is flexible and personalised, otherwise life events have a way of just taking over. A loss of self, coupled with a loss of perspective about what is happening, is not uncommon among carers in the early stages. Any book written about dementia will refer to carer burnout or carer distress or carer depression; this all too common scenario occurs because of the focus on the person with dementia and lack of attention to the carer in the early stages of dementia. Many people just go about their business and attempt to incorporate the person with dementia into their lives. When the needs of the person with dementia increase and the needs of the carer go unrealised, or unmet, an imbalance occurs. If basic needs are not met in any situation, there will be a stressed system. Something has to give, and inevitably it will be the carer's mental and physical health.

To avoid or minimise such circumstances a mental health care plan that is integrated with the needs of the person with dementia, as well as the needs of the family, offers a beginning that can be built upon as your circumstances change. This plan addresses concerns about the early stages of dementia. The needs of each family will be unique, but there tends to be an overall pattern. Separating the carer from the family and the person with dementia identifies what is exclusive to the carer and clearly identifies how the needs of the carer, the family and the person with dementia can so easily blur.

The psychosocial model in Table 15.1 depicts the separate and eclipsed needs of the carer, the person with dementia and the family.

The model demonstrates one way to show that the carer needs to manage changes that occur on many different levels simultaneously. Given that carers are depicted as having the most central role in caring for the person with dementia, health care workers can inadvertently create a paradoxical situation for the carer who is struggling to try to adapt, especially if they convey to the carer the impression that they need to provide care and self-care at the same time. This paradox is not often clearly stated, but the effects are clearly demonstrable in the numbers of carers that take anti-depressant medication as a way of coping and remaining resilient.

The word 'eclipsed' is used to demonstrate that the family and the person with dementia can be contained in one sphere and the carer in another sphere that is separate but which overlaps. Carers have responsibilities to the person with dementia that are different from the rest of the family. The family can take on some of the responsibilities some of the time, but ultimately overall care rests with the carer.

Carers are somehow expected to differentiate themselves and their needs from that of the person with dementia and the family, and how this is meant to be done is not often stated in the early stages of dementia. It tends to be an oversight until the carer is very stressed and seeks help, not for themselves, but for some aspect of providing care for the person with dementia.

The notion of being independent and self-sufficient—the silent coper—is hugely valued. The fact that depression will be the second leading cause of disability by the year 2020 and that we have recently set up a national institute of mental health clearly indicates that some unsubstantiated folklore needs reworking.

Table 15.1

Psychosocial Model

Changes to the family and the person with dementia	Changes for the carer
• Pre-diagnosis period; being diagnosed may take months to years; living with the unknown.	• Involved in the changes for the person with dementia and the diagnostic process.
• Selection of a carer usually comes from within the family.	• Carer role—volunteered or conscripted.
• Changes in roles and relationships in the family.	• Significance of relationship prior to diagnosis often needs to be reassessed in terms of the role that the person with dementia occupied and is now changed, e.g. breadwinner.
• Family adaptations—what support is going to be offered and by whom.	• Previous experience as a carer and its impact on the present situation, e.g. one parent with physical illness and now one with dementia.
• Beliefs about caring for parents.	• Adjustment and re-evaluations of time management skills if carer is still working and has children at home or maybe is caring for an adult child or grandchild.
• Education about dementia.	• Education about living with memory loss.
• Assessment of the current changes in the family and in the future, e.g. if parent is in another state or city.	• Understanding of how they see the current changes and the future.
	• Development of a health care plan for yourself.
• Equity and shared care—clarity of roles.	• Development of social network and supports.
• Grief and loss of the person as they had previously known them as a parent or spouse.	• Coping with ambiguous loss—person with dementia is physically present but intermittently psychologically absent.
• Conflicts between other family commitments—spouse, parent/s, kids, work, study, recreation.	• Assessment of personal strengths (resilience).
	• Assessment of personal faith and spiritual beliefs.
	• Ability to self-soothe, self-direct and self-regulate.
• Overall feeling of isolation—depression is very common for person with dementia in the early stages	• Differentiation of self—personal boundaries.
• Social death—coping with loss of friends and social activities.	• Re-investment in self and others on a different level.
• Adapting to the changes from the medical model to the psychosocial model.	• Advocacy—mastery.

An old dog can learn new tricks

The majority of carers are middle-aged or older and often feel that they are too old to take on new information and learn new skills. This is not usually stated as directly as this; rather, it may sound like, 'I am all right, don't worry about me, I will be fine'. Normal ageing, as a general rule, does not have a large impact on brain function. There will always be debate around this, but some people's best work was done in their seventies, eighties and nineties. George Frederick Handel wrote *Messiah* at fifty-six. Franz Joseph Haydn wrote *The Creation* at sixty-seven. Richard Wagner composed the opera *Parsifal* at sixty-nine. Martha Graham still choreographed in her nineties. Giuseppe Verdi wrote the opera *Falstaff* at eighty.[1] It is clear that these people continued to use their brain power well past some capricious or enforced age of retirement.

Scientists report that at birth we have about 100 billion neurons; that by our early twenties the brain has increased its mass threefold; that from here the brain drops in weight by 1 gram each year by natural causes—this equates to about 100 000 neurons each day of our lives; and that the average person loses about 10 per cent of his or her brain weight in a lifetime. Some of the causes of decreased brain function include medication, heart disease, prolonged grief, lack of exercise, lack of curiosity, lack of desire to learn new things, poor diet, depression, and alcohol.

Therefore, people can learn to do many things irrespective of age—especially where caring for oneself is concerned—and they can adjust to the needs of the person with dementia.

In one study a large number of carers revealed two major self-related categories: carer experience in terms of the emotions they felt, and the adjustments to caring that they had made. One carer described her feelings as:

> *A journey, and I guess that journey has taken us through the period of undiagnosed dementia, starting before the diagnosis, so*

at that stage we were pretty angry and, I guess, motivated by a lot of passion and frustration to actually get Mum diagnosed and to put it in [a little black box]... it was coming to terms with the diagnosis and having to learn by very difficult experience how to cope with the changes. I have not succeeded yet.

The common themes that were expressed by carers were loneliness, sadness, fear, anger, resentment, confusion, isolation, feelings of being trapped, loss of personal freedom, loss of personal space and disconnection from life. The significance of these themes shows that there was high emotional content, with many negative emotional feelings. The repetitiveness of the negativity expressed by many female carers strongly suggests that the carer owns or has internalised the problem. This means they believe the problems is theirs.

An alternative approach is to move from a position of adversity to one of resilience by learning how to self-care and, in the process, externalise the problems that surround the carer role. Problems, once externalised or clarified, are more manageable as this allows people to observe the problems impartially and offer management strategies for the problems.

The model of self-care proposed underlines the external adjustment and adaptations that are required, and possible ways to access the internal strengths that may be unrecognised when there is no distinction made between the role of the carer and the needs of the person with dementia.

SELF-CARE FOR CARERS

Step 1: Your physical health

Your physical health is connected to and controlled by many things: your genetic make-up, your attitude and your beliefs about health and what level of fitness you believe is right for you. Your beliefs about yourself in psychological terms were shaped many years ago, and over time you become what you believe. These beliefs are mostly uncon-scious and were formed in childhood in order to make sense of your world the best way you knew how. You don't generally separate your beliefs from your behaviour, and this is the main reason why fad diets and tough exercise routines do not last. Having external messages about how you should be or what you should do, will be at odds with your internal beliefs, and you can guess which one will have the strongest message and win every time.

The *New England Journal of Medicine* found that 'less that 10 per cent of physicians believed they were successful in helping patients change their behaviour. There is no magic pill to cure lethargy: you must be willing to make a few life-style changes for your health's sake.'[2]

When you reach mid-life you will 'know what you should do'; from time to time you will actually do it and feel good, but often your self-imposed régime is unsustainable. Knowing that you have an inner voice or a belief system allows you to examine whether the past beliefs are good for you now or have, in fact, passed their use-by date.

Many people feel guilty for not doing enough exercise on a reg-ular basis and this guilt is counter-productive. It serves no purpose and only leads to poor self-esteem. The cycle of motivation goes some-thing like this. You start off with high ideals and enthusiasm, then later you begin to feel some degree of anxiety about what you should be doing elsewhere. You reduce your exercise and finally it fades away, often leaving you both relieved and guilty. There will be another bout of motivation and the cycle continues. Look at the records of any gymnasium: the venue, the equipment, the ambience or the beautiful bodies will not sustain most people for great lengths of time. People will go to the gym with some mission such as losing weight for a wed-ding, achieve their goal then stop.

A health care plan designed specifically for your needs is essen-tially one that is temperate, gentle, self-nurturing and manageable. The 'shoulds' and 'musts' you repeatedly impose on yourself do not fit in with this model.

Most people know that women live longer than men and, as they age, half the population will have at least one chronic medical or psychiatric condition such as heart disease, arthritis, respiratory disease or vision problems. Being aware of the signs that something is not quite right, such as a change in bowel habits, dizzy spells or pain in some part of your body signals that there is a sick or stressed system that needs attention. Getting treatment early prevents further harm.

If you are ordered treatment, the directions must be adhered to. If the treatment does not appear satisfactory to you, go back and tell your local doctor, physiotherapist, dietitian or other health professional. With the plethora of treatments now available people tend to shop around and, in the process, only achieve part of the treatment required. Going back to the practitioner and discussing your concerns gives you the opportunity to have control over your treatment. Health professionals will modify treatments if they know. They are only people who are trying to offer a service, and to be fair they can't do anything about what they don't know.

You are a very important person, so regular check-ups with your doctor is good basic care. If your spouse has been the initiator of your medical care in the past, then this responsibility will now need to be resumed by you. Keeping medical appointments for yourself and the person with dementia can be time consuming but necessary.

With people now living well into their eighties and still wanting to stay in their own home and maintain a level of independence, your physical health is your best gold card. Being a carer adds unexpected responsibilities that can be managed if they are kept in perspective and you receive timely and appropriate support.

Step 2: Invest in yourself

The average age for men is 75.22 years and for women is 81.05 years. What is important is not how long you will live, but what the quality of that life will be. Being fit (age appropriate) and enjoying good health can be improved by a consistent level of movement, such as brisk walking for a specified time. Making a choice about how and when you move is best left up to you, as you are your best adviser, personal trainer and mentor. But move you must—on a regular basis.

Step 3: Your levels of stress

What triggers your stress? What reduces your stress? Develop a plan for your life that involves self-care. Learn alternative ways of living that provide you with a minimum of stress in your life while remaining connected to the person you are caring for.

Stress is a very individual experience: what stresses one person will not necessarily worry another. Stress is one word that definitely suffers from overuse in contemporary society. Do you remember your grandmother sitting down beside the mountains of washing, waiting for the copper to boil for the weekly Monday wash, saying that she felt stressed? Or her husband who had just handmilked seventy cows coming back to the house at dusk saying that he felt stressed? Imagine Captain Cook telling the first officer of the watch that he was leaving the ship and taking stress leave. Perhaps that is why people a century ago tended to live much shorter lives than we enjoy today. Maybe it was not all about disease and the lack of modern medicine; rather, it was feeling stressed but not having the word to describe the phenomena.

Stress is any constraining or impelling force that causes some significant modification of its form; it is physical, mental or emotional strain. Stress has a multitude of meanings, common among them the feeling of being out of control.

For carers, stress is the physiological and psychological response to a situation that, if unrelieved, causes tension affecting mental and physical health. Stress is also reported by people with dementia, especially in the early stages. The causes may be different but the effect is the same—the feeling of not being in control of a situation. The most positive aspect of stress is that it alerts you to the need to put up your hand and do something about it; for example, speak to someone about it and discuss options and strategies that will give you back some control.

Paying attention to how you feel, how the person with dementia states they are feeling, or observing their behaviour is the first step in the management of stress.

The physical signs and symptoms of stress include getting upset over an incident that is disproportionate to the event such as bursting into tears when the bathtub overflows, changes in weight, changed sleeping patterns, panic attacks, being short-tempered with people, raising your voice when no one around you has a hearing problem, headaches, increased alcohol intake, increased smoking, increased tiredness with a lack of spontaneity, feeling overwhelmed by the tasks that need to be routinely done and a loss of interest in sex.

In order to externalise stress you can do two things. Write down a list of issues or concerns that are bothering you. Don't be worried if you fill up a few A4 pages in the first round, because getting it out and down on paper allows you to see that it is real. Next, go back to the beginning of the list and put a feeling beside each item and, if possible, a reaction to that feeling. This activity separates an emotional response to an event from an objective situation, which needs a different strategy. For example, if the person with dementia has always done the cooking and suddenly you find that you are confronted by a cold kitchen each night at dinnertime, it will need a range of options and an individual plan to circumnavigate that problem.

One of the stressors about caring is that issues get all tumbled in together. It is difficult to see where one thing begins or ends, which leads to an emotional response from an already loaded system. Coping with the diagnosis and the changes to which you must adapt may have gone unnoticed by you. However, deep down below the level of the skin and into the microscopic level of the cells the anxiety has definitely registered. From your list you will begin to see a pattern emerging, showing things that trigger a response from you. Just note these down, as they will be one of the themes and will require some attention to minimise the effect that they are having upon you.

Breaking things down into manageable portions (even if on paper) allows you to move forward and develop a plan. The following is a list of things you can do when developing a plan to help reduce your stress.

- Take out a calendar and list all your 'must do' appointments for the month, for example, the doctor, the chemist, the hairdresser, work.
- Mark in the turnaround time, that is, how long it takes from getting yourself dressed and helping the person with dementia (if required), to driving to the appointment, having the appointment (include waiting time), driving home and parking the car.
- Next, put in your usual activities like shopping, cooking, cleaning, laundry, going to golf or bowls, attending a church service. Estimate the time that all these activities take.
- Include (if appropriate) child care duties, transportation, school work, supervision, afterschool activities.
- Next, put in family social engagements such as birthdays, weddings, gatherings for some necessary event.
- Insert activities that you might be involved with, such as cleaning or visiting your parents' home, taking a parent out for a drive or to the doctor, mowing the lawn (yours or someone else's), cleaning the pool.
- Include the family finances, as this is another task that does require at least monthly attention. You may need to visit your accountant or seek other help.

By this time the calendar will start to resemble a kaleidoscope, especially if you use different colours to separate what your tasks or responsibilities are and what you do for the person with dementia. You can put in tasks that are done in the home and those that require going out. This list does not involve accidents, repetitive questions, telephone calls, tradesman who do not show up, forgotten phone messages or family issues that regularly occur.

In our do-it-yourself (mythical) society, most of what needs to be done for the person with dementia will be assumed, often insidiously, by the carer. Prioritising what needs to go where in the early stages of dementia reduces the stress of attempting to do all the things that you have been able to do in the past.

Time management

You need to take stock of just what you are doing and how some tasks will need reallocation or elimination, such as doing tasks for other people that can be undertaken by a community service or by employing someone. Reviewing each of your activities will take time, but caring without becoming burnt out is all about good time management. Every business uses units of time and the measurement of outcomes to gauge its efficiency and potential profit. Part of the way that this is done is via downsizing, re-evaluation, retrenchment and restructuring, now normalised as part of the business activity of the world we live in. Closure of suburban branches of banks is an example; the fact that it inconvenienced many of its customers is neither here nor there. I am not suggesting that you will be as unfeeling, but you will need to give some consideration to where and how you can downsize your tasks in the future, if that is necessary for your situation.

When you downsize you will be able to afford time to self-care, which is the secret of good caring and will promote a calm environment for the person with dementia. It is not only your stress that you have to deal with, it is also the stress that the person with dementia experiences daily that can be heartbreaking to watch.

At the commencement of the Living with Memory Loss Program, people with dementia share with the group the frustrations that they experience on a daily basis when they are asked dumb questions regarding their memory. In the natural course of everyday speech you use many points of reference that require short-term memory, such as 'Did you see that film on TV last night? Wasn't it great when she …' or recounting fragments of the news in conversation. Not remembering recent events automatically moves the person with dementia outside the circle unless someone is paying attention and takes the time to include them in an update of the event. This calls for the carer to be continually relaying current information that will not be held by the person with dementia. Over time, the carer and others may not bother to keep the person with dementia in the conversation, as it becomes difficult unless the carer is well cared for. The person with dementia becomes more isolated and stigmatised.

Step 4: Understand your anger

In order to understand your anger, first know that it is only a feeling and that it is the flip side of love. 'To be angry with the right person to the right extent and at the right moment and with the right object and in the right way – that is not easy.'[3]

Anger is stress gone over the top or, to put it another way, anger is your response to a situation that is not what you want. It releases your breath, tension, anxiety and levels of frustration. It can even reduce you to tears. The downside is that anger only occasionally gets the results that you want, unless you are a very contained person who never demonstrates anger so an outburst shocks people around you and galvanises them into action that will somehow meet your needs.

People all have the capacity to feel anger, but it is what is done with the feeling that is worthy of note.[4] Repressed or silent anger has been linked to many major health problems like heart disease, immune system disorders, breast cancer, asthma, anorexia nervosa and white blood cell count abnormalities. Anger can be suppressed by internalising it, swallowing it, burying it, eating it, stuffing it or storing it within your body, causing obesity, stomach ulcers, bowel disorders and tension headaches.

Anger is energy, and holding on to it uses up emotional space that could be better used doing something more constructive or enjoyable. Some people are so used to suppressing their anger that they do not recognise the signs. Depression is a good example of unexpressed anger; all feelings are locked on the inside, because there is no safe place where the feeling behind the anger will be heard, understood and not taken personally. There are many words to describe anger that is expressed but very few to describe anger that is unexpressed or anger that remains on the inside.

Caring for a person with dementia can, at times, magnify aspects of your personality that you may prefer not to know existed, such as anger. It may not be caused by the person with dementia directly but could be related to an incident, such as a neighbour telling you for the fifth time in one week about the sufferer's behaviour in a derogatory manner while you stand there and smile. Or it could be triggered by the person with dementia driving in an unsafe manner and frightening you.

People with dementia can have an outburst of anger that is frightening and seemingly out of character, and can trigger your anger in response. Later on you may well feel ashamed or frightened by your behaviour. Learning to discharge your anger in appropriate ways is healthy. Emotional release, for some people, occurs in a variety of ways, such as a good sexual relationship, doing energising sporting activities, hitting a golf or tennis ball, power walking, dancing, exercise, screaming into a pillow—anything that works and does not hurt anyone else. Anger in the form of yelling and screaming at other people does not change anything; it only leaves you feeling exhausted and having to cope with additional issues such as the reaction, criticism or emotional response of other people who have witnessed your anger.

Anger and love in marital relationships

If the person you are caring for has been a source of love, contentedness and a best friend you will be dealing with a complexity of issues within yourself. You will have survived the period of coming to terms with the reality that another person will not be available to supply all of your needs. Covertly or overtly, this stage requires a lot of push and pull, where couples try to shape their partner into what they want them to be. You have learnt to manage your life together and see your partner as having needs that are separate to yours while remaining connected. You will be in the invisible process of slowly reverting back to being a single person. This awareness often strikes people at moments when they are relaxed, vulnerable, tired or stressed.

> *I was reading this funny part in a book and I turned to Harry and said, 'Listen to this'. I began reading and started laughing and when I looked up after I had finished he was just staring out of the window. He didn't get the funny side. This feeling hit me right in the middle of my chest—I felt so desperately alone at that moment.*

Anger and love are inexorably linked. Pleasure and pain both come from the one source—yourself. You can get upset or angry with a person and still love them. Being angry continually causes harm to yourself if there is no one there to hold or soothe you when the explosion subsides. The anger is most often caused by not having your needs met in the same way—it is not necessarily what the person with dementia is doing. It is having to do more for yourself, emotionally and functionally.

Adapting to the changes in your life, primarily, is an internal, self-reflective process. Learning what and how to manage life with someone with dementia is a cognitive task, but having a bank of literature on the table is not enough when your tears are falling. Learning how to process these emotions takes time and support. Support can come via a support group, individual or couple counselling, your family or a circle of supportive friends. What has proven to be helpful is connecting with people who are in a similar situation, as it provides input from other people who are negotiating similar uncharted terrain. A friend can support, but the input is not as effective.

16 Resilience

THE FATHER OF WESTERN MEDICINE, HIPPOCRATES, ONCE SAID that the human body can only be understood as a whole. Having harmony with the three dimensions—mind, body and spirit—creates a feeling of peace that most people have experienced perhaps only fleetingly during their lifetime. In today's frenetic world the notion of harmony or peace is often presented to consumers as something that they can buy such as a new car or a holiday, something that will take them away from their home and give them something different. Relaxation is often understood as doing nothing, stopping, having no responsibilities. This artificial relaxation can come at a high financial cost. Caring for someone with dementia will necessitate the carer finding harmony with themselves on a regular basis. This chapter outlines a few ideas for personal harmony or a connectedness with yourself that is achievable and affordable in both money and time.

The strategies outlined for gaining personal harmony include the person with dementia as much as possible. The person with dementia can be involved when they are supported appropriately. Maintaining the person with dementia's integrity as a human being is paramount to the notion of support and care.

The notion of resilience is largely related to a person having certain individual personal resources that will help them cope or respond to life's difficulties, seeing changes as either a challenge or an opportunity for personal growth. It is an important personality resource that might enable individuals to adapt and negotiate their lives under changing conditions. Researchers have identified that resilient people are meaningfully engaged with the world.[1] Their positive and energetic approach to life is grounded in a sense of mastery within a wide range of life's domains.

People included in the vast body of current research on resilience include children from war-torn countries; prisoners of war; families where a parent is mentally ill, emotionally abusive, criminal or neglectful; and women who have sustained emotional and physical violence for many years. Women need to be especially resilient as they watch the generation they have loved and respected and counted on for emotional support leave them and the children they have raised test their wings and fly from the nest. This is a time when new relationships need to be formed and new activities need to be found, as the child-related involvement of the past is no longer necessary. This is a time for self-renewal and self-investment that will sustain them as they face challenges and life issues that require negotiation.

Carers of a person with dementia will in time come to terms with the fact that the person with dementia will no longer think and act normally and will readjust their lifestyle accordingly—they will let go of the need to struggle to be in control. They will consider the fact that they need to do what they can and then let others help when necessary.

Developing resilience

Most people are aware of difficulties or troubles before they occur, and they are motivated to make things better by searching for solutions,

Table 16.1

Resiliency definition and concepts[2]

Resiliency	Definition/concepts
Insight	The mental habit of asking searching questions and giving honest answers. This subscale includes the concepts: Sensing: reading signals from other people Knowing: identifying the source of the problem, and Understanding: trying to figure out how things work for self and others.
Independence	The right to safe boundaries between yourself and significant others. This subscale includes the concepts: Distancing: being able to emotionally distance from people who pull you around, and Separating: knowing when to separate from bad relationships.
Relationships	Developing and maintaining intimate and fulfilling ties with other people. This subscale includes the concepts: Recruiting: perceived ability to select healthy supportive relationships, to start new relationships, and Attaching: to maintain healthy relationships.
Initiative	Determination to master oneself and one's environment. This subscale includes the concepts: Problem solving: creative problem solving/enjoyment of figuring out how things work; and Generating: generating constructive activities.
Creativity and Humour	Safe harbours of the imagination where you can take refuge and rearrange the details of your life to your own pleasing. This subscale includes the concepts: Creative thinking: creativity/divergent thinking Creating to express feelings: being able to use creativity to forget pain, using creativity to express emotions, and Humour: using humour to reduce tension or make a bad situation better.
Morality	Knowing what is right and wrong and being willing to stand up for those beliefs. This subscale includes the concepts: Valuing: knowing what is right and wrong and being willing to take risks for those beliefs; and Helping others: liking to help other people.
General resiliency	This subscale was included to assess: Persistence: persistence at working through difficulties, and Flexibility: confidence that they can make the most of bad situations.

learning new ways of coping and reaching out for support. Resilience is a strength that can be learnt or developed if some thought is given to the process. While every person is different and no two situations are identical, some carers will be more susceptible to stress and some individuals will be more resilient than others. Everyone will have their limits. Knowing the key issues which need to be addressed to attain some level of resilience can be helpful.

Having a framework offers the carer or the counsellor a model that can be used as a reference point when you are feeling off centre in your life. What others have found is that when they lose perspective in one area of their lives, it skews all the other aspects accordingly. If you are feeling alone and unsupported this will take up a lot of emotional energy, with the result that the other areas where you can have some balance are neglected.

Being de-energised, in general, is counter-productive to creative or divergent thinking. For many carers, focusing on yourself requires a philosophical shift in beliefs that takes time. As long as the main points in Table 16.1 are being covered, a notion of resilience will start to occur automatically.

How would you know it you were moving forward? Certainly by the fact that you have a reduction in the amount and length of time that you are feeling negative emotions like anger, frustration or despair or are more concerned about things outside your self disproportionate to what is occurring in your inner world. This, incidentally, is about the only thing most of us can control. A wise carer once said: 'When I finally realised that he was not going to change and it was going to be all up to me, that is when I began to feel better.'

The body and the mind

Taking care of yourself is a decision that doesn't come automatically to most people. Being overcommitted to something or someone or overworking is more believable than being involved in self-care. Many people often feel that all the good things they are supposed to do for themselves amounts to 'high personal maintenance', but did you think that when you were rearing your children, studying, doing the second job or still in the workforce and juggling care? Caring for yourself is often way down on the 'to do' list. The fact that you are a 'human being' and not 'human doing' gets overlooked as you strive to do more or take on that extra little chore each day.

Many carers suffer from sleep deprivation which goes unnoticed until there is an uproar over an event that in other circumstances would have been experienced differently for both the carer and the person with dementia. Understanding and experiencing your body as more than its physical form takes some creative thinking.

Suggested here are some aids that, while not new, can be a starting point for gaining a balance for the mind, body and spirit. Things that a person can do to become fully conscious or totally aware 'if life is to be fully lived, but not substitutes for the living of life itself, with its demands, complexities, hurts and joys'.[3] As well as those outlined here you can also try remedial massage, reflexology and facials.

Relaxation

The breath is the only thing that connects you to this world. Unless there is a problem with your respiratory or cardiac system or you run out of puff from overexertion your breathing is hardly noticed. Using your breath to focus your attention is one way to begin to relax. Just notice your breathing cycle, in and out, in and out, inspiration and expiration.

Take the phone off the hook for ten minutes. Soften the lights or draw the curtains or blinds. Put on your favourite meditation music if you choose. Sit in an upright chair with your hands unclasped in your lap. With your eyes open, focus on a spot across the room. Focus your attention on your breathing—just be aware of it. Take five deep breaths to expel the old stale air. Keep focusing on your breath and start to slow down the time between each breath. Close your eyes and listen for six things or sounds that you can hear. Focus your attention on six things that you can feel.

Move your attention to your heart and imagine it as having four sections that open and close smoothly and rhythmically. With each breath, imagine your heart opening and closing like a large sea anemone that is opening and closing, floating silently through the clear blue waters of a calm Atlantic Ocean. Watch it float, softly, gently, just being there at peace with the watery world. The only sounds are the movement of the fins of the fish as they move around in the water.

Keep your breathing even and relaxed—just observe. You don't have to do anything; just be in the moment. If any thoughts come into your mind, brush them aside and refocus on your breathing.

Feel your shoulders soften and your spine become heavy on the back of your chair. You may hear the sound of a whale singing somewhere far off in the distance. Just be, just sit, just watch for a moment in time when you are totally connected to yourself. Your heart rate and your breathing will slow, your blood pressure will drop and your body will be at rest.

When you are ready, allow yourself time to come back into the room for the transition into a more active state. Wriggle your fingers and toes. Open your eyes and stay sitting for a few minutes while you reconnect to your surroundings. Take a nice long stretch either sitting or standing.

Have a positive affirmation somewhere near you to read after your relaxation/meditation, then it will be the first thought that enters your mind in its refreshed state of consciousness. Try these positive affirmations.

> *Happiness is not a destination; it is a method of life. When the heart weeps for what it has lost the spirit laughs for what it has found. In the centre of difficulty lies opportunity (Albert Einstein).*

You cannot reheat a soufflé (L. Bott).

The difference between a flower and a weed is a judgment.

When you have mastered these simple steps for yourself you can guide the person with dementia through this relaxation process by softly and slowly going through each step. This method has been used many times in groups for people with dementia and it works. An additional benefit is that this activity is something that can be done by anyone in the family, as a settling technique for the person with dementia after they have been feeling stressed. Often they do not have the initiative to commence meditation themselves, but with the right environment they will follow your voice in this guided meditation. It does not require any special equipment or professional person. Twice a day would be the ideal; once a day is okay also.

Creating the right environment for relaxation can be done physically or via your imagination. It is stopping to take heed or notice of your breathing that is the key element. People with dementia respond to relaxation exercises, as the activity is slow. Use music, subdued lighting, comfortable clothes and an upright position in a comfortable chair with your feet placed on the floor uncrossed. Put your hands in your lap without touching. Laying on the floor is an option, but there is the danger of falling asleep.

A relaxing bath

Busy people frequently opt for a shower, as it is efficient and quick and allows more time to do more things. Relaxing in a bathtub of warm scented water with the phone off the hook takes time and is more leisurely; you can immerse all of your body in warm, caressing water which soothes tired limbs. An additional treat is to use bath bombs. Scented balls that dissolved in the bath add another dimension of pleasure; some even have petals in them. Scented water with floating petals: imagine!

Music

Music provides a wonderful source of relaxation. Select your favourite piece of music and sit or lie down with your eyes closed and listen. This will help to reduce the tension and stress that builds up in your body daily. While you are listening you can tense and relax your fingers and toes and your abdominal muscles.

Aromatherapy

Aromatherapy is an old art that uses concentrated essential oils to promote or restore emotional health and wellbeing. The oils evaporate when exposed to the air. Essential oils can be used daily as well as in your regular bathing. Add six to ten drops of essential oils to your bathtub and soak for twenty to thirty minutes. You may choose to light a candle and burn another oil in your diffuser.

Humour

Laughter is a great stress reliever. Hire a funny video or watch something truly funny on the TV. Listen to a radio program that you enjoy.

Tai chi

Tai chi has been used for centuries as a method of relaxation for the mind and body. People of all ages and states of physical health can enjoy this either in a class or through use of a video tape in the comfort of your own loungeroom.

Slow motion is a powerful method to develop dynamic relaxation. Doing any movement slowly allows you to notice and begin to be aware of the tension in your muscles. Focus your attention on the body and the breath.

Tai Chi is non-competitive. You can go at your own pace or even slower. This can be difficult for some people, as they are used to doing things quickly. Slowing down draws your attention to your body, and to where you are holding tension.

Walking

Walking is excellent. Making time for your walk is probably more difficult than the walk itself, but establishing a routine for you and the person with dementia will reap great benefits. Instead of saying 'Do you want to go for a walk?' you might say, 'Come on, let's go for a walk together.' You be the initiator—people with early stage dementia often have great difficulty getting started. It is not laziness, it is part of the brain damage. Walking is an activity that you can enjoy together for a long time.

Regular health check-ups

Your health is very important, so seeing your own doctor every six to twelve months is good practice. Monitoring the medications for the person with dementia, especially if they have other medications as well as the anti-dementia drugs, takes time and attention, so it is easy to forget your own health needs. It is understandable that the regular medical reviews for the sufferer's special needs can make going to your own doctor less important; however, you have certain responsibilities for your own health.

Keeping a journal

Paying attention to your thoughts and feelings, dreams and daily emotional experiences assists in keeping you mentally fit. Your psyche or mind is as much a part of you as any other organ in your body and holds aspects of both your conscious and unconscious life. If you are unaware of your psyche or pay scant attention to what you are experiencing it is very likely that you will project it on to others.

Projection is the process by which one's own traits, emotions and dispositions are ascribed to others. There are parts of yourself that you don't want to know about so you deny they exist which protects you from the anxiety that your beliefs or feelings may create. Not reflecting upon what is happening to you on the inside (or in your mind and feelings) makes projection much more likely. As a result, it is much more probable that you will become reactive to life's events rather than proactive, to attain the much more desirable sense of mastery in your life.

One way of keeping track of your interior world is to keep a journal, which is different from keeping a diary. A diary contains details of daily life such as appointments, events, meetings and birthdays, whereas a journal is a personal time capsule that can be used for personal growth or as a tool in therapy. Writing about personal problems, feelings and anxieties can help clear your mind. Once it is on paper, it externalises the problem and allows for more objective thinking about the problem for yourself or reflection with another person. Orr, a psychologist at the University of New South Wales' Counselling Service, believes that 'writing and exploring your concerns helps prevent worries from permeating every waking minute of the day...an individual can dedicate time to working on a problem and not exhaust themselves worrying'.[4]

Journal entries can be used to observe patterns in your behaviour and triggers for your reactions. Many things can go into a journal each day and, as you cultivate the practice, you can then write about the day's psychological episodes; for example, you can review an angry scene that occurred with someone on that day or reflect upon something that touched you when you met someone or when you saw or heard something beautiful. A journal is a medium for holding your thoughts, private fears, fantasies, dreams, wild urges and black thoughts (the shadow side, that part of you that you do not want to own). Even thoughts such as 'I wish that so and so were not here' serve to defuse those thoughts and feelings that are too private for some to share with other people for fear of being criticised.

Connecting with your unconscious is paying attention to those thoughts that just drift through your mind when you are in a relaxed state or doing another activity such as walking or taking a bath. Creative pursuits in other areas of your life such as ideas for a holiday, drawing or painting, taking a course, singing or writing are more likely to occur when you remain connected to both your inner and outer worlds.

Keeping a journal is a short cut to gaining valuable insight, one of the hallmarks of resilience. When perused over time, it gives rise to the sense of mastery or a sense of connectedness with life, which is the goal that most people either consciously or unconsciously aspire to. Put another way, journal writing creates an energy field enabling you to connect with the resources to practise the wisdom of: 'If opportunity does not knock, build a door. Make your happiness happen.'

A cautionary note: a journal rattles your soul. It needs to be protected. Even in the most trusting families curiosity is part of human nature. You need to be able to write with total honesty or you will do yourself a disservice. A thought that someone might read your journal is counterproductive to the whole exercise. Margaret Knorr in *New Woman* suggests that you can:

- Find the nicest book that you are comfortable with—the best note book.
- Use a special pen, one that writes smoothly, and don't use this pen for anything else.
- Use a different-coloured ink from what you normally use. This aids the capturing of your thoughts or moments which otherwise may be lost.
- Create a special place, a haven, for your writing.
- Write at the same time each day. Writing is like any other skill—it takes practice. Artists and musicians practise regularly.[5]

A life story

When people cannot identify themselves as they did in the past it is helpful for them and others to know where they came from. A biographical memoir or life story is something that can be done in the early stages of dementia as a joint exercise with the person with dementia and a friend, carer or family. I have started to do this 'remembering' exercise in the memory loss groups which I run. People with dementia can lose the ability to write or express themselves clearly in the present moment, but oral history tends to comes naturally. It is the minute details that make up the exquisite fabric of people's lives and create the individual story. Often this oral history takes place of its own accord in the first or second meeting; it sets a contextual framework for others in the group to relate to others, rather than being just another person with dementia. These sessions offer us a very different view of the person sitting beside us. It is one of the most powerful events in these groups.

Many of us who work with confused elderly people would agree that our knowledge of the illness is inclined to be somewhat sparse. If these patients are seen as the sum total of the problems then the outlook is bleak. We need to see the person behind the dementia.

A life story offers individualisation for the person with dementia as well as the carer, as the recording of their life helps us to realise that they are not the family or the carer's persona. They have walked their own path, and irrespective of what we may think about proprietorial rights or ownership of that person in the present, they are uniquely individual.

A life story is not about fixing past hurts or solving current ones, but it can be used for the family or others to have insight into a person's life. It can be used as a memory jogger for the person with dementia and later on for other carers to help deliver more personalised care, especially in understanding explanations for some behaviours that may be occurring today. When creating a life story book, key points to consider including are:

- The name preferred.
- The place of birth.
- The events around birth; for example, Henry Lawson was born in a tent near a railway line in the middle of a raging storm.
- The date of birth.
- The first language.

- Names of parents and grandparents if known.
- Dates of parents' deaths.
- The names of brothers and sisters.
- Schooling and educational background.
- When they stopped school and why.
- First paid employment and the story of how that came about—was it by choice or necessity.
- War service.
- Marriage date and circumstances. If female, describe the wedding outfit including colour and fabric. Any funny happenings on the day. Where did they go for a honeymoon?
- Places that they have lived in and why.
- Greatest achievements.
- Favourite animal or pet.
- Hobbies and sports they were involved in.
- Best job they ever had.
- The names of special friends.
- Greatest loves—film stars, books, places, country, music, theatre, TV or radio.
- Favourite activities in the past and present.

This is a broad outline of a person's life. Interviewing is best done when the person is fresh in the morning, and it is best to go at the pace set by the person with dementia. Sometimes they will be full of information, anecdotes and stories from the past; at other times the information will be less forthcoming. The richness will be found in the details recounted; for example, a person who has been a fighter pilot in the war may want to discuss aeroplanes, or a dancer may tell of a performance. If possible, ask them what was the song or music or the colour of their costumes. Nothing can restore the memory, but having a mosaic of the highlights of a person's life is a wonderful historical record for the family to know where they came from and what role their ancestors played in the wider picture of their contemporary society. Autobiographies and biographies of famous people sit on the shelves in libraries—your person with dementia is your connection to both the past, the present and the future.

Spirituality

As Plato said: 'You ought not to attempt to cure the body without the soul… For this is the great error of our day in the treatment of the human body, that physicians separate the soul from the body.' A person's spirituality and faith is inexorably linked on some level. A model of faith 'involves holding onto oneself and not giving in to fear when things do not seem to be going to one's liking: holding onto to oneself for security involves coping with disappointment without losing one's sense of direction in life.'[6]

Faith is at the heart of the mystery of human life. It enables a person to perceive what is real—to see through the appearances of things and people. The philosopher Kierkegaard wrote, 'Man only begins to exist in faith.'[7] By this he meant that to exist as a human being is to live with faith. Faith involves firm belief in something or someone beyond ourselves. Faith takes the human person beyond the confines of belief based on scientific evidence. If there is evidence, we simply believe whatever is evident as demonstrated or 'proved'; for example, $2+2=4$. Faith takes us beyond the limits of reason and leads us to surrender to the mystery that lies within being and existence itself.

On a simplistic level, faith is wishing or wanting to have life the way that we want it to be. Hanging on to this view is counterproductive, as it reduces one's capacity significantly to be able to see the larger picture and the possibilities of a wonderment that is happening all around. As the pop group the Rolling Stones sang: 'You can't always get what you want, but if you try, sometimes you just might find you get what you need!'

My research of carer resilience revealed that faith in some higher power provided the greatest source of comfort when caring for people with dementia. As one carer reported:

> When Mum has a little lie down so do I, and when she goes for a walk so do I. It is not a problem. It won't be long before I will not be able to walk with her. I am sustained by my faith—there is nothing that is sent to us that we can't handle. I have always believed this so I was prepared in a way. After all, this is just another part of the joys and sorrows of life.

Following on from this revelation about the impact of faith on caring, I interviewed a good friend who I consider lives her life with faith.

Could you give me some of your thoughts on your faith from a practical point of view?
Faith allows us to live each day as a gift. We trust that life will always bring us what we need to become our best selves, and that we will be given the wherewithal to deal with whatever comes our way. In fact, we believe that we can learn from all that happens in our own lives and the world around us.

How is that actually done?
When we live with faith we learn to let go of fear, which causes us to want to control so much of life; and so we gradually feel less isolated within ourselves and from life around us. As faith is tested through each day's experiences, we find ourselves stronger in spirit. So we are invited to move beyond childhood needs, while at the same time to live with a deepening sense of responsibility to sustain the spirit of community.

But what about the really hard time in life?
While the inevitable times of pain and suffering in life will test us to the limit of our being, even to the point of feeling abandonment by God, it is through faith that we will find the courage to stay with the

journey through the valley of darkness until the light of a new dawn breaks through, and we can move on to the next stage of life. Those who live through such times with faith emerge richer and more compassionate people.

What does faith teach you?
It is faith that teaches us to trust that all will be well—all manner of things will be well. Faith nourishes a sense of being in communion with others. It enables us to see with the inner eye of love and seek out the points of connection that nourish the fragile environment that provides the soil for genuine forgiveness and reconciliation—in families and among peoples of all cultures.

It sounds so simple when said like that but I am curious to know how you stay connected to your faith, which I understand goes far beyond a person's belief in something, some higher power.
Faith becomes a belief in oneself as a manifestation of the goodness of God, not an appeal as an insignificant creature to a greater power.

From this interview I learned that the previous carer's view of faith had in fact surpassed the notion of mastery to being in the realms of surrender. No longer did she struggle with the concepts of faith; she had totally internalised her faith and it had become part of her world view or her philosophy of life and all that it encompassed, including her role as a carer.

Aboriginal philosophy

In Western society the spiritual dimension of the human condition often gets overlooked in the process of people learning about dementia. While researching for her Ph.D, Deborah Forrest noticed nurses who were descendants of Cherokee Indians speaking and singing to patients who were no longer fully conscious or had any notion of personal identity. They treated these people and referred to them as if they were young and healthy. Intrigued by this depth of care, she discovered their belief that the spirit is central to all life.[8]

Miriam-Rose Ungunmerr talks about the Aboriginal quality of *dadirri*, which she describes as that inner, deep listening from 'the deep spring that is inside us'—listening to nature, and listening to the people's stories that have been passed down and enacted in ceremonies through the centuries. If truly lived, *dadirri* brings a deep awareness and a way of knowing that the Aboriginal person does not necessarily articulate in words.

This spirituality underpins the Aboriginal respect for life as it presents itself, in nature and in the community of each tribe. The anthropologist Dr Stanner wrote that the 'Aboriginal religion was probably one of the least material-minded, and most life-minded of any of which we have knowledge'.[9] Stanner said that the Aboriginal philosophy was one of 'assent to life'. Life is expressed by living faithful to the myths and beliefs of the ancestors, passed down in story and ceremony, and lived in the present according to custom and tribal law. Contrary to the Western way of thinking, the Aboriginal philosophy of life does not perceive change as inherent to life. Things must remain as they have been from the beginning. This has a profound effect on the way life is lived out in the day-to-day events within families and communities. For example, the community will accept a person's way of living or behaviour with a simple comment, 'That's him'. Even if a person acted a bit differently or strangely, this would most often be interpreted as 'just part of them'.

Aboriginal people are by nature most accepting of other people— they have a high level of tolerance for people's behaviour. Mental and physical disorders may not be seen as separate, and may be covered by the term 'sickness'. However, distinctions are drawn between sickness and disturbed behaviour or 'madness'. It is only when a person causes great shame or disruption to family or community that there will be a shift in the community's innate spirit of tolerance.

Appendix I

Statistics about dementia

- At the beginning of the 21st century it is predicted that more than 34 million people worldwide will develop Alzheimer's disease by 2020.
- Dementia is a syndrome caused by a range of illnesses. Most are currently incurable and cause progressive, irreversible brain damage. They include Alzheimer's disease (the most common cause), vascular disease, front lobe dementia, Lewy Body disease and AIDS.[1]
- Symptoms of dementia can include memory loss, difficulties with language, judgment and insight, failure to recognise people, disorientation, mood changes, hallucinations, delusions and the gradual loss of ability to perform all tasks of daily living.[2]
- Over 700 000 people in the UK have dementia. More than half of those have Alzheimer's disease. 33 000 people in Ireland have Alzheimer's disease.
- One in twenty people over the age of sixty-five will develop dementia. This compares to one in five people over the age of eighty.

- 55 per cent of people with dementia will develop Alzheimer's disease.
- The Alzheimer's Society estimates that there are about 18 500 people between thirty and sixty-four with Alzheimer's disease.
- The average length of time a person will live with dementia is ten to fourteen years.
- Dementia is the fourth biggest killer of adults after heart disease, cancer and diseases of the respiratory system.
- Age and family history are the two major risk factors for Alzheimer's disease.

Appendix II

Diagnostic criteria for dementia of the Alzheimer's type—taken from the *Diagnostic and Statistical Manual of Mental Disorders*[1]

A. The development of multiple cognitive defects manifested by both
   1. Memory impairment (impaired ability to learn new information or to recall previously learned information)
   2. One (or more) of the following cognitive disturbances:
      (a) aphasia (language disturbance)
      (b) apraxia (impaired ability to carry out motor activities despite intact motor function)
      (c) angosia (failure to recognise or identify objects despite intact sensory function)
      (d) disturbance in executive functioning (i.e. planning, organising, sequencing, abstracting)

B. The cognitive deficits in Criteria A1 and A2 each cause significant impairment in social or occupational functioning and represent a significant decline from a previous level of functioning.

C. The course is characterised by gradual onset and continuing cognitive decline.

D. The cognitive deficits in Criteria A1 and A2 are not due to any of the following:
   1. other central nervous system conditions that cause progressive deficits in memory and cognition (e.g. cerebrovascular disease, Parkinson's disease, Huntington's disease, subdural haematoma, normal-pressure hydrocephalus, brain tumour)

2. systemic conditions that are known to cause dementia (e.g. hypothyroidism, vitamin B12 or folic acid deficiency, niacin deficiency, hypocalcaemia, neurosyphilis, HIV infection)
3. substance-induced conditions

E. The deficits do not occur exclusively during the course of a delirium.

F. The disturbance is not better accounted for by another Axis I disorder (e.g. major depressive disorder, schizophrenia).

Appendix III

Folstein Mini Mental State Examination[1]

Max score	Score	
		Orientation
5	( )	What is the (year), (season), (date), (month), (day).
5	( )	Where are we: (state), (city), (what part of the city—e.g., near the sea, eastern suburbs), (which community centre), (floor).
		Registration
3	( )	Ask if you can test the individual's memory. Name 3 objects (e.g., apple, table, penny) taking 1 second to say each one. Then ask the individual to repeat the names of all 3 objects. Give 1 point for each correct answer. After this, repeat the object names until all 3 are learned (up to 6 trials). Number of trials needed:
		Attention and Calculation
5	( )	Spell 'world' backwards. Give 1 point for each letter that is in the right place (e.g., DLROW=5, DLORW=3).
		Alternatively, do serial 7s. Ask the individual to count backwards from 100 in blocks of 7 (i.e., 93, 86, 79, 72, 65). Stop after 5 subtractions. Give 1 point for each correct answer. If one answer is incorrect (e.g., 92) but the following answer is 7 less than the previous answer (i.e., 85), count the second answer as being correct.

Recall

3   (   )   Ask for the 3 objects repeated above. Give 1 point for each correct object.

Language

2   (   )   Point to a pencil and ask the individual to name this object (1 point). Do the same thing with a wristwatch (1 point).

1   (   )   Ask the individual to repeat the following: 'No if, and no buts' (1 point). Allow only one trial.

3   (   )   Give the individual a piece of blank white paper and ask him or her to follow a 3-stage command: 'Take the paper in your right hand, fold it in half and put it on the floor' (1 point for each part that is correctly followed).

1   (   )   Show the individual the 'CLOSE YOUR EYES' message on the following page (but not the pentagons yet). Ask him or her to read the message and do what it says (give 1 point if the individual actually closes his or her eyes).

1   (   )   Ask the individual to write a sentence on a blank piece of paper. The sentence must contain a subject and a verb, and must be sensible. Punctuation and grammar are not important (1 point).

1   (   )   Show the individual the pentagons on the following page and ask him or her to copy the design exactly as it is (1 point). All 10 angles need to be present and the two shapes must intersect to score 1 point. Tremor and rotation are ignored.

_____   **Total Score**

CLOSE YOUR EYES

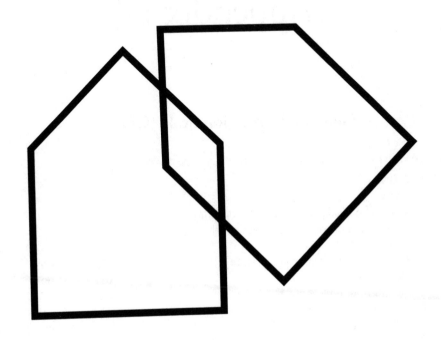

Appendix IV

Geriatric Depression Scale (GDS)[1]

Choose the best answer for how you felt this past week
CIRCLE ONE

*1.	Are you basically satisfied with your life?	yes	NO
2.	Have you dropped many of your activities and interests?	YES	no
3.	Do you feel that your life is empty?	YES	no
4.	Do you often get bored?	YES	no
*5.	Are you hopeful about the future?	yes	NO
6.	Are you bothered by thoughts you can't get out of your head?	YES	no
*7.	Are you in good spirits most of the time?	yes	NO
8.	Are you afraid that something bad is going to happen to you?	YES	no
*9.	Do you feel happy most of the time?	yes	NO
10.	Do you often feel helpless?	YES	no
11.	Do you often get restless and fidgety?	YES	no
12.	Do you prefer to stay at home, rather than going out and doing new things?	YES	no
13.	Do you frequently worry about the future?	YES	no
14.	Do you feel you have more problems with memory than most?	YES	no
*15.	Do you think it is wonderful to be alive now?	yes	NO
16.	Do you often feel downhearted and blue?	YES	no
17.	Do you often feel pretty worthless the way you are now?	YES	no
18.	Do you worry a lot about the past?	YES	no

*19. Do you find life very exciting?	yes	NO
20. Is it hard for you to get started on new projects?	YES	no
*21. Do you feel full of energy?	yes	NO
22. Do you feel that your situation is hopeless?	YES	no
23. Do you think that most people are better off than you are?	YES	NO
24. Do you frequently get upset over little things?	YES	no
25. Do you frequently feel like crying?	YES	no
26. Do you have trouble concentrating?	YES	no
*27. Do you enjoy getting up in the morning?	yes	NO
28. Do you prefer to avoid social gatherings?	YES	no
*29. Is it easy for you to make decisions?	yes	NO
*30. Is your mind as clear as it used to be?	yes	NO

* Appropriate (non-depressed) answers = yes, all others = no or count number of CAPITALISED (depressed) answers

Score:

Norms	(Number of depressed answers)
Normal	5+/-4
Mildly depressed	15+/-6
Very depressed	23+/-5

Notes

1. Introduction

1 D. Cohen and C. Eisdorfer (1986) in L.K. Wright, *Alzheimer's Disease and Marriage—An Intimate Account*. Sage, Newbury Park, 1993, p. 3.
2 Dementia Fact Sheet, Alzheimer's Association of New South Wales, 2000.
3 A.S. Reber, *The Dictionary of Psychology*. Penguin, London, 1985, p. 448.

2. Pre-diagnosis

1 www.alzheimers.com/health_library/diagnosis/diagnosis_02_warning.html
2 C. Boden, *Is it Alzheimer's? Warning Signs You Should Know.* Reprinted with permission from the National Alzheimer's Association of the United States, 1998.
3 H. Gruetzner, *Alzheimer's: A Caregiver's Guide and Source Book*. Wiley, New York, 1992, p. 17.
4 D. Weddington, *Early Stage Alzheimer's Care: A Guide for Community-based Programs*. Springer Publishing Company, New York, 1994, p. 19.

3. Being diagnosed

1 D. Kuhn, *Alzheimer's Early Stages: First Steps in Caring and Treatment*. Hunter House, California, 1999.
2 L.A. Klata et al, *Incorrect Diagnosis of Alzheimer's Disease*. Archives of Neurology, Chicago, 1996.
3 M.F. Folstein, S.E. Folstein & P.R. McHugh, 'Mini Mental State: A practical method for grading the cognitive state of patients for the clinician' in *Journal of Psychiatric Research*, 1975, no. 12, pp. 189–98.
4 I. McDowall & C. Newell, *Measuring Health: A Guide to Rating Scales and Questionnaires*. 2nd edition, OUP, New York, 1996.
5 G. Small, *Alzheimer's Disease—Early Signs*. The Health Report, Radio National, 4 December 2000. See also the website http://abc.net./au/rn/talks/8.30/ helthrpt/stories/s220499.htm

6   HCF Special Report, *Alzheimer's Disease*. Custom Publishing Group, Australia, 1998, pp. 6–7.

7   G. Andrews, *Management of Mental Disorders. Treatment Protocol Project*. 3rd edition, vol. 1, World Health Organisation, Competitive Edge Graphics, Sydney, 2000, p. 27.

8   Fact sheet from the Alzheimer's Association of the United States, figure 2, 'Telling the Patient, Family and Friends'. Reprinted with permission.

9   H. Wilkinson & M. Downs, 'The effect of being told the diagnosis of dementia from the perspective of the person with dementia'. Mental Health Foundation news release, 30 July 1999. See also the website http:/www.mentalhealth. org.uk/pressl.htm

10 American Psychiatric Association, *Diagnostic and Statistical Manual of Mental Disorders*. 4th edition, Washington DC, 1994.

11 A.J. McCutcheson, 'Changing the Philosophy of Dementia Assessment: A new service for the assessment and management of problems related to dementia'. Alzheimer's Association of Australia, 1999.

4. Behavioural changes

1   http.//www.ama-assn.org/insight/gen_hlth/atlas/newatlas/brainlob.htm

2   G. Laborde, *Fine Tune Your Brain: When everything's going right and what to do when it isn't*. Syntony Publishing, Palo Alto, California, 1988, p. 99.

3   Alzheimer's Association of New South Wales, 2000.

5. Drug treatments

1   M. Nash, 'The New Science of Alzheimer' in *Time* magazine, 17 July 2001.

2   P. Davies (1970) in J. Rogers, *Candle and Darkness. Current Research in Alzheimer's Disease*. Sun Health Research Institute, Arizona, 1996, p. 63.

3   P.J. Howard, *The Owner's Manual for the Brain*. Leornian Press, Texas, 1994, p. 37.

4   Alzheimer's Disease Society, 'Appraisal for Drugs for Alzheimer's Disease', London, 1999, p.15.

5   The preceding information was supplied by courtesy of the Alzheimer's Disease Society, Gordon House, 10 Greencoat Place, London SW1. Telephone 0171 306 0606; fax 0171 306 0808. They also have an Alzheimer's help line on 0845 3000 0336 that is available from 8 am to 6 pm Monday to Friday.

6   H. Brodarty, D. Ames, et al. 'Pharmacological treatment of cognitive deficits in Alzheimer's disease' in *Medical Journal of Australia*, 2001, vol. 175, pp. 324–29.

7   Forstl, *Clinical Issues*.

8   H. Brodarty, D. Ames, et al. 'Pharmacological treatment of cognitive deficits in Alzheimer's disease' in *Medical Journal of Australia*, 2001, vol. 175, pp. 324–29.

9   The Melbourne *Age*, 3 August 2000.

10 C. Masters, The Mental Health Research Institute of Victoria, Alzheimer's Disease Division, 2000. See also the website http://www.mhri.edu.au/add/

11 H. Gruetzner, *Alzheimer's: A Caregiver's Guide and Source Book.* Wiley, New York, 1992, p. 6.

12 C. Boden, *Who Will I Be When I Die?* HarperCollins Religious Publishers, Melbourne, 1998, p. 156.

13 D. Kuhn, *Alzheimer's Early Stages: First Steps in Caring and Treatment.* Hunter House, California, 1999, p. 68.

14 R. Ochs, 'Conclusion uncertain', http://www.newsday.com/news/health/altmedp2.htm#gingko

6. A rite of passage

1 K. Doka & R. Aber (eds), *Disenfranchised Grief—Recognising Hidden Sorrow.* Lexington Books, Massachusetts, 1989, p. 188.

2 ibid., p. 6.

3 J. Kelly, 'The Ageing Male Homosexual: Myth and Reality' in *The Gerontologist,* vol. 17, 1997, pp. 238–332.

4 E.M. Brody, S.J. Litvin, C. Hoffman & M.H. Kleban, 'Differential Effects of Daughter's Marital Status on Their Parent Care Experiences' in *The Gerontologist,* vol. 25, 1992, p. 59.

5 D. Weddington, *Early Stage Alzheimer's Care.* Springer Publishing Company, New York, 1994, p. 19

6 G. Burrows, 'The Darkness Within' in the *Sydney Morning Herald,* 17 July 1999.

7 P. Ackerman, 'War is Health for a Nation of Moaners' in the *Sydney Morning Herald,* 5 August 1999.

8 J. Finch & D. Groves, *A Labour of Love: Women, Work and Caring.* Routledge & Kegan Paul, London, 1980. Also, Rosenmayer & Kockeis (1963) in *A Labour of Love,* p. 118.

9 Alzheimer's Disease International Fact Sheet 3, April 1999.

7. Beyond the patient: partners, family and friends

1 L. Boscolo, G. Cecchin, L. Hoffman & P. Penn, *Milan Systemic Family Therapy: Conversations in theory and practice.* Basic Books, New York, 1987, p. 4.

2 M. Yapko, *Hand-me-down Blues.* Golden Books, New York, 1999, p. 49.

3 D.G. Gallagher-Thompson & H.M. DeVries, 'Coping with frustration—Classes: Development and preliminary outcomes with women who care for relatives with dementia' in *The Gerontologist,* vol. 34, 1994, pp. 548–52.

8. The Living with Memory Loss Program

1 R. Yale, *Developing Support Groups for Individuals with Early-Stage Alzheimer's Disease.* Health Professions Press, Baltimore, London, Toronto, Sydney, 1995.

2   'Sharing Dementia Care', the Alzheimer's Association of New South Wales, Winter 2000.

3   D.F. McGowin, *Living in the Labyrinth*. Delta Books, Bantam Doubleday, New York, 1993.

4   T. Kitwood, 'Discover the person, not the disease' in *Journal of Dementia Care*, vol. 1, no. 1, November/December 1993 in M. Goldsmith, *Hearing the Voice of People with Dementia—Opportunities and Obstacles*. Jessica Kingsley, London, 1996, p. 23.

5   E. Peach & Duff, 'Mutual support groups: A response to the early and often forgotten stage of dementia' in *Practice*, vol. 6, 2000, p.149.

6   C. Bryden, P. McGrath & M. Bryden, 'Support groups in the ACT for people in early to moderate stage dementia: Valuing the person with dementia for whom they are now', National Conference of the Alzheimer's Association, 21–25 September 1999, p. 223.

7   W. Lustbader, 'Counting Kindness: The Dilemmas of Dependency' in D. Kuhn, *Alzheimer's Early Stages: First Steps in Caring and Treatment*. Hunter House, California, 1999.

8   M. Longhurst, *The Beginner's Guide to Retirement*. Hodder Headline, Sydney, 2000.

9   P. Cerexhe, *Before and After Retirement*. Choice Books, Marrickville, Sydney, 2000.

10 'Power of Attorney in New South Wales: A Guide', Land and property information at http://www.lto.nsw.gov.au/publications/info_kits/pofa-02.html

11 Seniors information sheet, 'Wills and Living Wills' at http://www.add.nsw.gov.au/sis/sis_wills.htm

12 D. Kuhn, *Early Stage Alzheimer's Disease*. Hunter House, California, 2000, p. 181.

13 A. Berndt, 'Driving Assessment and Rehabilitation Service', National Conference of the Alzheimer's Association at the School of Occupational Therapy, University of South Australia, 21–25 September 1999, p. 79.

14 M.A. Steinberg & M.A. Peel, 'Veterans' Health', National Conference of the Alzheimer's Association, 22–23 July 1999, p. 84.

15 Sleep Apnea Research Association in *Apnea News*, December 2000, p. 5.

16 E. Gray, 'Promaco Conventions', National Conference of the Alzheimer's Association, 21–25 September 2000, p. 141.

17 A. de Mello, *The Prayer of the Frog*. Gujarat Sahitya, Prakash, Anand, India, 1988, p. 27.

18 N.L. Mace & P.V. Rabins, *The 36 Hour Day*. Johns Hopkins University Press, Baltimore, 1991, p. 216.

9. The family

1   W. McLeod, *New Collins Dictionary and Thesaurus*. Collins, London, 1987, p. 351.

2   S.R. Sauber et al, *Dictionary of Family Psychology and Family Therapy*. Sage Publications, Newbury Park, 1993, pp. 134, 142.

3　Fischer & Toronto in *Family Caregivers: Disability, Illness and Ageing*, (ed.) H. Schofield et al, Allen & Unwin, Sydney, 1998.

4　G. Dalley, 'Ideologies of Caring' in *Family Caregivers: Disability, Illness and Ageing*, (ed.) H. Schofield et al, Allen & Unwin, Sydney, 1998.

5　J.R. Twigg, K. Aitken and C. Perring, 'Carers and Services: A Review of Research', Social Policy Research Unit, London, Her Majesty's Stationery Office, 1990.

6　G. Dalley, *Ideologies of Caring*. Macmillan Education, United Kingdom, 1988.

7　B. Carter & M. Goldrick, *The Changing Family Life Cycle: A Framework for Family Therapy*. 2nd edition, Allyn & Bacon, Boston, 1989, p. 15.

8　J.M. Nankervis, S. Block, B.M. Murphy & H.E. Herman, 'A Classification of Family Carers' Problems as Described by Counsellors' in *Journal of Family Studies*, vol. no. 2, October 1997, pp. 169–82.

9　T. Kitwood, The Psychology of Caring, interview by Professor Anthony Clare for the BBC Radio program 'All in the Mind' recorded in *Journal of Dementia Care*, July/August 1996, p. 11.

10　J. Gilliard, 'Ripples of Stress Across the Generations' in *Journal of Dementia Care*, July/August 1996, pp. 17, 18.

11　B. Carter & M. Goldrick, *The Changing Family Life Cycle*, p. 323.

12　B. David & P. Birtles, 'Money Matters—The Hidden Costs for Families Caring for Patients with Early Onset Dementia', Alzheimer's Association National Conference Papers, 1997, p. 109.

13　W.J. Worden, *Grief Counselling and Grief Therapy: A handbook for the mental health practitioner*. 2nd edition, Springer Publishing Company, New York, 1991.

14　T.A. Rando, 'A Comprehensive Analysis of Anticipatory Grief: Perspectives, processes, promises and problems' in T.A. Rando (ed.), *Loss and Anticipatory Grief*, Lexington Books, Massachusetts, 1986, pp. 3–38.

15　K. Gilbert, 'Grief in a Family Context' on http://www.indiana.edu/~hperf558

16　C. Revson, *Oxford Dictionary of Modern Quotations*. Oxford University Press, Oxford, 1998.

17　W.J. Worden, *Grief Counselling and Grief Therapy*.

18　L. Malet, 'The Wages of Sin: Coping with Cognitive Impairment. Some Family Dynamics and Helping Role' in *Journal of Gerontological Social Work*, vol. 4 (3/4), spring/summer, 1982.

19　F. Wilks, *Intelligent Emotion*. William Heinemann, London, 1999, p. 154.

20　W.F. Lynch, *Images of Hope*. Notre Dame Press, Helicon, Baltimore, 1987, pp. 32, 33.

10. The family system

1　M. Yapko, *Hand-me-down Blues*. Golden Books, New York, 1999, p. 49.

11. Caring for the carer

1 Y. Wells & O. Over, 'Institutional Placement of a Dementing Spouse: the Influence of Appraisal Coping Strategies and Social Supports' in *Australian Journal of Psychology*, vol. 50, no. 22, 1998, pp. 100–105.

2 A. Clare, 'The Psychology of Caring' in *Journal of Dementia Care*, July/August 1996, p. 11

3 A. Kaplan, 'Caring for the Caregivers: Family Interventions and Alzheimer's Disease' in *Psychiatric Times*, vol. xv, issue 9, September 1998. See also http://www.mhsource.com/pt/p989047.html

4 S. Cauchi, 'GPs treating more depression' in the Melbourne *Age*, 30 October 1999. See http://www.theage.com.au/news/19991030/A14866-1999Oct29.html#top

5 M. Yapko, *Hand-me-down Blues*. Golden Books, New York, 1999, p. 49.

6 K. Gibran, *The Prophet*. Heinemann, London, 1926, p. 26.

12. Hidden loss

1 'Ambiguous Loss and Disenfranchised Grief: Grief in a Family Context' on http://www.indiana.edu/~hperf558/summer98/ambiguous.html

2 P. Boss, 'Ambiguity: A Factor in Family Stress Management' on http://www.extension.umnedu/distribution/familydevelopment/DE2469.html

3 ibid.

4 S.R. Sauber, et al, *The Dictionary of Family Psychology and Family Therapy*. 2nd edition, Sage Publications, Newbury Park, 1993, pp. 38, 104, 339.

5 L. Parrott, 'The Control Freak' on http:www.psychjournal.com/Interviews-2000/October00_Parrott2.htm

13. Attachment and non-attachment

1 D. Winicott, 'Hate in the counter transference' in *Through Pediatrics to Psychoanalysis*. Hogarth, London, 1958. Also in J. Holmes, *Attachment, Intimacy and Autonomy*. Aronson, Northvale, 1996, p. 205.

2 E.J. Bourne, *The Anxiety and Phobia Workbook*. New Harbinger Publishers, California, 1990, p. 3.

3 J. Holmes, *Attachment, Intimacy and Autonomy*, p. 84.

4 B.M.L Miesen, 'Attachment Theory and Dementia' in G. Jones & B.M.L. Miesen (eds), *Caregiving and Dementia: Research and Applications*. Routledge, London, 1993.

14. Counselling

1 P. Boss, *Ambiguous Loss*. Harvard University Press, Cambridge, 2000, p. 30.

2 P. Watzlawick, Weakland & Fisch (1974) in T. Bobes & B. Rothman, *The Crowded Bed*, W.W. Norton & Company, New York, 1998, p. 189.

3   T. Bobes & B. Rothman, *The Crowded Bed*. W.W. Norton & Company, New York, 1998, p. 190.
4   ibid., p. 191.

15. Looking after yourself

1   P.J. Howard, *The Owner's Manual for the Brain*. Leornian Press, Austin, Texas, 1994, p. 60.
2   C. Meyers, *Walking*. Random House, Australia, 1992, p. 13.
3   F. Wilks, *Intelligent Emotion*. Heinemann, United Kingdon, 1998, p. 74.
4   J. Pennebaker (1990), 'Opening Up: The healing power of confiding in others' in J. Lee (ed.), *Facing the Fire. Experiencing and Expressing Anger Appropriately*. Bantam Books, New York, 1993, p. 6.

16. Resilience

1   J.H. Block & J. Block, 'The role of ego-control and ego-resiliency in the organization of behaviour' in W.A. Collins (ed.), Minnesota Symposia on Child Psychology. Hillsdale, New Jersey, 1980, pp. 39–101.
2   S.J. Wolin & S. Wolin, *The Resilient Self: How survivors of Troubled Families Rise Above Adversity*. Villard Books, 1993.
3   J. Stanford, *Healing and Wholeness*. Paulist Press, New York, 1997, p. 120.
4   F. Orr, 'The write stuff' in *New Woman*, vol. 62, 1996, pp 62–65.
5   M. Knorr, 'Do you journal?' in www.geocities.com/Wellsley/Garden/5347
6   B. Suzanne, www.plato-dialogues.org/plato.htm
7   S. Kierkergaard in J. Stanford (ed.), *Healing and Wholeness*. Paulist Press, New York, 1997.
8   D. Forrest, *Symphony of Spirits*. St. Martins Press, New York, 2000, pp. 47 and 79.
9   Dr. Stanner referenced in Miriam-Rose Ungunmeer, text of talk given at the International liturgical conference in Tasmania, 1998.

Appendix I

1   Dementia fact sheet, Alzheimer's Association of New South Wales, 2000.
2   ibid.

Appendix II

1   DSM–1V, *Diagnostic and Statistical Manual of Mental Disorders*. 4th edition, Washington DC, p. 146.

Appendix III

1   M.F. Folstein, S.E. Folstein & P.R. McHugh, 'Mini Mental State: A practical method for grading the cognitive state of patients for the clinician' in *Journal of Psychiatric Research*, 1975, no. 12, pp. 189–98.

Appendix IV

1   J.A. Yesavage, T.L. Brink, T.L. Rose, et al. Development and validation of a geriatric depression rating scale: a preliminary report. *J Psych Res.* vol. 17, 1983, p. 27. J.I. Sheikh & J.A. Yesavage Geriatric Depression Scale: recent evidence and development of a shorter version. *Clin Gerontol,* vol. 5, 1986, pp. 165–72.

Contacts

The Alzheimer Society of Ireland

www.alzheimer.ie

Internet Resources

Age Action Ireland

www.ageaction.ie

Age Action Ireland is the national independent organisation on ageing and older people. It acts as a network of organisations and individuals including older people and carers of older people and as a development agency promoting better policies and services for older people and an ageing society.

Alzheimer's Disease International

www.alz.co.uk

ADI is an umbrella group of 60 Alzheimer associations throughout the world. Each of our members is the national Alzheimer association in their country who support people with dementia and their families.

Alzheimer Europe

www.alzheimer-europe.org

Alzheimer Europe is a Non-Governmental Organisation aimed at raising awareness of all forms of dementia through coordination and cooperation between Alzheimer and related disorders organisations in Europe, as well as organising support to the sufferers of the disease and their carers.

Alzheimer's Society – UK

www.alzheimers.org.uk

The Alzheimer's Society is the leading care and research charity for people with Alzheimer's disease and other forms of dementia, their families and carers.

Department of Health and Children
www.doh.ie
The Department of Health and Children has overall responsibility for the development of health policy and for the planning of health services.

Dementia Services Information and Development Centre
www.dementia.ie
The Centre aims to promote an awareness of dementia, establish and maintain a database on dementia services in Ireland, provide education and training to practitioners working in the field and conduct and support local and international research and evaluation.

Alzheimer's Society
Local support

The Society has a network of branches in England, Wales and Northern Ireland.

England

Bedfordshire
www.alzheimers.org.uk/**NorthBeds**

Berkshire
www.alzheimers.org.uk/**Slough**

Cambridgeshire
www.alzheimers.org.uk/**Fenland&Marshland**
www.alzheimers.org.uk/**Peterborough**

Cheshire
www.alzheimers.org.uk/**EllesmerePort&Neston**

Cumbria
www.alzheimers.org.uk/**Carlisle**
www.alzheimers.org.uk/**SouthLakeland**
www.alzheimers.org.uk/**WestCumbria**

County Durham
www.alzheimers.org.uk/**Darlington**
http://www.alzheimers-durham.org.uk

Essex
www.alzheimers.org.uk/**Harlow**

Hampshire
www.alzheimers.org.uk/**Portsmouth**
www.alzheimers.org.uk/**Winchester**

Herefordshire
>www.alzheimers.org.uk/Herefordshire

Hertfordshire
>www.alzheimers.org.uk/Dacorum
>www.alzheimers.org.uk/NorthHerts&Stevenage
>www.alzheimers.org.uk/StAlbans
>www.alzheimers.org.uk/Watford
>www.alzheimers.org.uk/WelwynHatfield

Kent
>www.alzheimers.org.uk/WestKent

Leicestershire
>www.alzheimers.org.uk/Leicestershire&Rutland

Lincolnshire
>www.alzheimers.org.uk/Grantham
>www.alzheimers.org.uk/SouthLincolnshire

London
>www.alzheimers.org.uk/Barnet
>www.alzheimers.org.uk/Bromley
>www.alzheimers.org.uk/Redbridge
>www.alzheimers.org.uk/Southwark
>www.alzheimers.org.uk/WalthamForest

Norfolk
>www.alzheimers.org.uk/Norwich

Northamptonshire
>www.alzheimers.org.uk/SouthNorthants

Northumberland
>www.alzheimers.org.uk/Berwick

Nottinghamshire
>www.alzheimers.org.uk/Nottingham

Shropshire
>http://www.salz.org.uk

Somerset
>www.alzheimers.org.uk/Mid-Somerset
>www.alzheimers.org.uk/NorthSomerset

Suffolk
>www.alzheimers.org.uk/Ipswich
>www.alzheimers.org.uk/WestSuffolk

Surrey
>www.alzheimers.org.uk/Dorking
>www.alzheimers.org.uk/EastSurrey
>www.alzheimers.org.uk/Haslemere
>www.alzheimers.org.uk/Woking

Susssex (East)
    www.alzheimers.org.uk/**Brighton**
Tyne and Wear
    www.alzheimers.org.uk/**Newcastle**
    www.alzheimers.org.uk/**Sunderland**
Warwickshire
    www.alzheimers.org.uk/**SouthWarwickshire**
West Midlands
    www.alzheimers.org.uk/**Birmingham**
    www.alzheimers.org.uk/**Coventry**
    www.alzheimers.org.uk/**Dudley**
    www.alzheimers.org.uk/**Walsall**
    www.alzheimers.org.uk/**Wolverhampton**
Worcestershire
    www.alzheimers.org.uk/**Worcester**
    www.alzheimers.org.uk/**WyreForest**
Yorkshire (North)
    www.alzheimers.org.uk/**York**
    www.alzheimers.org.uk/**Craven** (Skipton)
Yorkshire (West)
    www.alzheimers.org.uk/**Bradford**
    www.alzheimers.org.uk/**Huddersfield**

Wales

www.alzheimers.org.uk/**Blackwood**
www.alzheimers.org.uk/**NWWales**

Northern Ireland

www.alzheimers.org.uk/**NIreland/NDA** (North Down and Ards)
www.alzheimers.org.uk/**NIreland/Newry**

Useful websites

Carers Association of Australia:
    www.carers.asn.au/index.html

Carers Association of Australia (Dementia page):
    www.carers.asn.au/dementia.html

The Caregiver's S.E.A. (Support & Education for Alzheimer's diseases):
    www.neuro-oas.mgh.harvard.edu/sea/index.html

Alzheimer's Association (USA):
    www.alz.org/

Alzheimer's Disease Society (UK):
    www.alzheimers.org.uk/framestart.htm
Alzheimer_Disease_Research_Center (ADRC)'s Alzheimer Page:
    www.adrc.wustl.edu/ALZHEIMER
Dementia Page:
    www.dementia.ion.ucl.ac.uk/
Caregiving Online:
    www.caregiving.com/
Caregivers Helping Other Caregivers:
    www.isl.net/~hoffcomp/
Partners Program of Excellence in Alzheimer's:
    www.neuro-oas.mgh.harvard.edu/alzheimers/
Alzheimer Web:
    www.werple.mira.net.au/~dhs/ad.html- OR:
    www.dsmallpc2.path.unimelb.edu.au/ad.html
Alzheimer's—Dr John S. Carman Research:
    www.carmanresearch.com/alzheimers.html
Alzwell Caregiver Page:
    www.alzwell.com/
The Alzheimer's Disease Web Page:
    www.med-amsa.bu.edu/Alzheimer/home.html
Alzheimer's Information for Children and Adolescents:
    www.alz.org/us/rtrlchil.htm
Aphasia (Word-finding & other communication problems):
    www.aphasia.org/

Links to other Alzheimer's websites and resources

Mental Health Matters (Alzheimer page):
    www.mental-health-matters.com/alzheimer.html
Comprehensive Services on Aging (COPSA) Institute for Alzheimer's Disease and Related Disorders:
    www.rwja.umdnj.edu/~coyne/copsa.html
Alzheimer's Links:
    www.ar-msj.demon.co.uk/links.htm

'ALZHEIMER' email discussion group:
To join the discussion group, send an email to: <majordomo@wubios.wustl.edu> with the following command written in your email message: 'subscribe alzheimer' (An email reply will request confirmation of intent to join.) Further information about this discussion group is available at: Alzheimer Disease Research Center (ADRC)'s Alzheimer Page www.adrc.wustl.edu/alzheimer

Index

Aboriginal philosophy, 237
abstract thinking, problems with, 14
accommodation, 107, 116
acetylcholine, 60–66
activities to improve brain function, 108
adjustment disorders, 156–157
Aged Care Assessment Teams (ACAT), 48
agnosia, 55
AIDS, 73, 163, 238
alternative therapies, 68–70
Alzheimer, Alois, 3
Alzheimer's Association, 27, 50
  client, definition, 6
  contact details, 256–258
  educational material, 41, 50
  inviting people to attend group, 41
  Living with Memory Loss Program
    see Living with Memory Loss
    Program
  referral to, 38, 47
  services, 50
  support from, 39, 42
Alzheimer's disease, 2, 3, 16
  diagnostic criteria, 47, 240–241
  early warning signs, 11–16

  likelihood of developing, 3, 28
anger, 137, 151, 217–220
anticholinesterase drugs, 61–66
anti-inflammatory drugs, 69
anti-oxidants, 69, 70
apraxia, 55
Aricept, 61, 64, 65
aromatherapy, 69, 228
assessment
  diagnosis, for, 31–32
  drug treatment, before, 62
attachment, 172–178

basic testing for dementia, 29
behavioural changes, 14–15, 18–22, 51–58
  brain degeneration, links to, 55–57
  depression, 24–25
  drugs, effect of, 62
  early warning signs, 14–15
  pre-diagnosis period, 18–20, 84–85
  recognising symptoms, 26
  younger onset dementia, 20–22
Binswanger's disease, 16
Borson, Soo, 155
Boss, Dr P, 164
Bowen, Dr Murray, 148, 166, 173

brain
    atrophy, 35, 36
    behavioural effects of degeneration,
        55–56
    function, 53–58
    lobes, 54–58
    maintaining function, 108–109, 209
    neuronal structure, 60
    parts of, 53–58
brain scans, 34–36
Bryden, Christine, 69, 97

carer *see also* family
    adjustment disorders, 156–157
    adjustment process, 134–139
    anger, 137, 151, 217–220
    asking for help, 41
    attachment, 172–178
    caring for, 151–161
    changes for, 208
    coming to terms with problem, 52
    counselling, 154–155, 179–201
    definition, 5–6
    depression, 153, 157–159, 218
    effect of social attitudes on, 2,
        74–75
    equal involvement in caring, 85–89
    expanding knowledge about
        dementia, 113–115
    family caregiver, 129–133
    fear and anxiety, 175–177
    financial aid, 140–141
    future, planning for, 115–117
    hardship, 138–139
    health, 153, 210–213, 229
    informing others, 41–44
    intimacy and sexuality, 117–120
    journal, keeping, 229–231
    Living with Memory Loss Program
        for, 93–94, 110–120
    looking after self, 115
    meaning of caregiving, 129–133
    mental health care plan, 206–208
    model of care, 81–82

    needs of, 82, 151–161
    non-attachment, 177–178
    only child, 195–201
    physical health, 210–213
    primary carer, 129
    profile of average carer, 76, 131
    relaxation, 225–228
    resilience, 221–237
    resources available for, 46
    selection of, 129–134
    self-care, 210–220, 224–239
    stress, 153, 159–161, 213–216
    support for, 82, 85–89, 151–161
    time management, 216–217
CAT scan, 35, 36
Cerexhe, Peter, 106, 107
characteristics of dementia, 2, 3, 5,
    238
    diagnostic criteria, 47, 240–241
    early warning signs, 11–16
    pre-diagnosis period, 11–29
children, effect on, 18–19, 133–134
cholineacetyltransferase, 60–61
Cognex, 61, 66
Cognitive Dementia and Memory
    Services, 48
cognitive testing, 33
communication, improving, 103–105
comprehension
    brain part controlling, 55, 57
    cognitive testing, 33
connection, 56
    brain part controlling, 56
contacts, 256–260
controlling behaviour, 171, 188–189
counselling/therapy, 154–155, 179–201
    couple, 154, 156, 188
    family, 147–150, 156, 187–195
    objectives, 185, 186, 192, 197
    only child, 195–201
    systemic, 148, 179, 197
couples
    anger and love, 218–220

carer partner *see* carer
counselling, 154, 156, 186
intimacy and sexuality, 117–120
creativity, 223
Creutzfeldt-Jakob disease, 16
CT scan, 35, 36

Davies, Dr Peter, 60
de Leon, Dr, 35
depression, 15, 18, 20, 24–25, 77–78
behavioural changes, 24
carers, 153, 157–159, 218
distinguished from dementia, 24–25
major/clinical, 25
minor/reactive, 25
physical problems contributing, 24
reaction to dementia, 77–78
reversible dementia, cause of, 17
sexuality and, 118
signs and symptoms, 25
diagnosis, 30–46
acceptance of, 91–93
assessment, 31–32
diagnostic criteria, 47, 240–241
effect of receiving, 73
informing family and friends, 39,
41–44
informing person with dementia,
39–41
initial consultation by GP, 32–37
results, getting, 37–39
treatment options, 47–50
value of getting, 30
differentiation, 170–171
disorientation, 13–14
cognitive testing, 33
doctor *see* general practitioner; medical
specialist
doctor and specialist management plan,
47–48
Doka, Prof Kenneth, 73
donezepil hydrochloride, 65
Downs, Dr Murna, 44
driving, 109

drug treatments, 59–70
anticholinesterase drugs, 61–66
anti-inflammatory drugs, 69
Aricept, 61, 64, 65
assessment for, 62
benefits, 64–65
carers, advice about, 114
clinical trials, 67–68
Cognex, 61, 66
commencing treatment, 62
cost, 140
donezepil hydrochloride, 65
effect, 64
Exelon, 61, 64, 65
galantamine, 61, 65
hormone replacement therapy, 69
how drugs work, 63–64
monitoring progress, 62–63, 229
obtaining, 66–67
reminyl, 61, 65
rivastigmine, 65
side effects, 65–66
tacrine hydrochloride, 61, 66
DSM-IV, 47, 240–241

early stage dementia, definition, 5, 11
early warning signs, 11–16
abstract thinking, problems with, 14
behavioural changes, 14–15
difficulty with familiar tasks, 13
disorientation, 13–14
initiative, loss of, 15
judgment, loss of, 14
language problems, 13
misplacing things, 14
mood changes, 14–15
over age 65, 22–24
personality changes, 15
recent memory loss, 12–13
recognising, 26
younger onset dementia, 20–22
EEG scan, 34
Exelon, 61, 64, 65

faith, 234–237
familiar tasks, difficulty with, 13
  practical strategies for coping,
    102–103
family *see also* carer
  adjustment process, 134–139
  anger, 137, 176
  attachments, 172–178
  boundaries, 167–169
  children, effect on, 18–19, 133–134
  collaborative approach, 43
  concept of, 75–76
  contributions of relationships, 82
  controlling behaviour, 171
  counselling/therapy, 147–150, 156,
    187–195
  denial by, 27, 136–137
  differentiation, 170–171
  effect on, 18–19, 74–75, 139–141
  equal involvement, 85–89
  escaping, 137–138
  fear and anxiety, 175–177
  fear of inheriting disease, 138
  financial adjustment, 139
  genogram, 165–166, 173, 174
  grief and loss, 72–74, 141–146,
    162–171
  hardship, 138–139
  importance of, 81, 82, 125–146
  inability to recognise, 55
  informing, 39, 41–44
  lack of support from, 42–43
  members, definition, 6
  only child, 195–201
  pre-diagnosis period, 18–20, 84–85
  relationship changes, 103–105,
    125–127
  roles, changes in, 126, 128
  secrets, 136
  seeking help, 26
  selection of carer, 129–134
  structure, changes to, 127–128
  system, 82–84, 147–150

  unequal involvement, 86–87
family history of dementia, 28, 34
family therapy, 147–150, 156,
    187–195
finances
  adjustment, 139
  effect on, 139–140
  financial aid, 140–141
  planning, 106, 116
  services, 140–141
focusing on the positive, 103
Folstein Mini-Mental State
    Examination (MMSE), 33, 62, 66,
    100, 242–243
Forrest, Deborah, 236
frequently asked questions, 26–29
front lobe dementia, 238
frontal lobe, 56–57
  behaviours affected, 55–56
future, planning for, 105–107
  accommodation, 107, 116
  carers, 115–117
  finances, 106, 116
  guardianship, 107, 117
  power of attorney, 106, 117, 190
  will, 107, 117

galantamine, 61, 65
general paresis, 16
genogram, 165–166, 173, 174
general practitioner
  basic testing by, 29
  changing doctors, 38
  doctor and specialist management
    plan, 47–48
  initial consultation by, 32–37
  role of, 29, 31
  test results, giving, 37–39
  typical questions asked by, 32
  writing down questions for, 29
Geriatric Depression Scale (GDS), 33,
    246–247
ginkgo biloba, 69–70
grief and loss, 72–74, 79, 162–171

ambiguous loss, 163
anticipatory, 142, 162
coping with, 145–146
family members, 141–146
hidden loss, 73, 162–171
relocation, 142–143
working towards hope, 143–146
guardianship, 107, 117

Hayley, Jay, 148
hope, 143–146
hormone replacement therapy, 69
humour, 110, 194, 223, 228
Huntington's disease, 16

incidence of dementia in Australia, 2,
3, 238–239
informing people
diagnosis, after, 39–46
family and friends, 39, 41–44
initial concerns, 27, 28
lack of support, 42–43
non-disclosure, 39, 42, 43, 44
person with dementia, 39–41, 44–45
right to know, 45–46
initiative
brain part controlling, 56
loss of, as early sign, 15
resilience, developing, 223
insight
brain part controlling, 55
cognitive testing, 33
resilience, developing, 223
intimacy, 78, 117–120
irreversible dementias, 16

journal, keeping, 229–231
judgment, loss of, 14, 57
brain part controlling, 55, 57
cognitive testing, 33

Kitwood, Dr Tom, 96, 154
Kuru, 16

language
brain part controlling, 55, 57
cognitive testing, 33
problems as early sign, 13
laughter, 110, 194, 223, 228
Lewy Body disease, 64, 238
life story, 231–234
likelihood of developing dementia, 3,
238–239
family history, 28, 34
living alone, 78–79
Living with Memory Loss Program,
90–122
acceptance of diagnosis, 91–93
agenda, 100–110
basis, 93–94
carer support groups, 93–94,
110–120
courses, 90
criteria for joining, 99
feedback from groups, 121–122
joining a group, 98–101
MMSE to assess impairment, 100
ongoing groups, 120
operation of program, 94–98
origins, 97–98
preliminary interview, 99–100
sufferer support groups, 93–94,
101–110
treating whole person, 95–96
Longhurst, Michael, 106
loss see grief and loss

media portrayal, 1
medical examination
cognitive testing, 33
initial consultation by GP, 32–37
medical history, 34
pathology tests, 34
physical examination, 34
results, getting, 37–39

scans, 34–36
medical specialist
    assessment by, 31
    doctor and specialist management
        plan, 47–48
    referral to, 29
memory, 3–5
    brain part controlling, 55, 57
    long-term, 4
    recent memory loss, 12–13
    short-term, 3–4
    what is, 3–5
mental health care plan, 206–208
Minuchin, Salvadore, 148
misplacing things, 14
MMSE, 33, 62, 66, 100, 242–243
mood changes, 14–15, 18–20
    drugs, effect of, 62
    early warning signs, 14–15
    pre-diagnosis period, 18–20
morality, 223
MRI scan, 35
multi-infarct dementia, 16
music, 228

non-disclosure, 39, 42, 43, 44
    right to know, 45–46
non-steroidal anti-inflammatory drugs,
    69

parietal lobe, 57
    behaviours affected, 55–56
Parkinson's disease, 16
partner *see* carer; couples; family
pathology tests, 34
patient
    definition, 6
    informing of diagnosis, 39–41
    right to know, 45–46
perseveration, 56
    brain part controlling, 56
persistent forgetting, 28
personality changes, 15
personhood, concept of, 96

PET scan, 35
physical examination, 34
physical problems contributing, 17, 22,
    24
Pick's disease, 16
power of attorney, 106, 117, 190
practical strategies for coping, 101–103
pre-diagnosis period, 11–29
    behaviour, 18–20, 84–85
psychotherapy, 156

recent memory loss, 12–13
recognition
    brain part controlling, 55, 57
regulation, 56
    brain part controlling, 56
relationships *see also* family
    changes, 103–105, 125–127
    contributions of, 82
    resilience, developing, 223
relaxation, 225–228
Reminyl, 61, 65
resilience, 221–237
    concepts, 223
    developing, 222–224
resources available, 46
reversible dementias, 16, 17
rivastigmine, 65

Satir, Virginia, 148
seeking help, 26
    family members, 26–27
    reluctance, dealing with, 27
Seloke, Dr Dennis, 59
sexuality, 117–120
shame, 77–78
Small, Prof Gary, 35
social attitudes, 1, 76–77
    effect of, 72–75
spatial awareness
    brain part controlling, 55, 57
    problems, as early sign, 13–14
specialised care centres, 48–49
spirituality, 234–237

Stanner, Dr, 237
statistics about dementia, 238–239
stress, 159–161
    carer, 153, 156, 159–161, 213–216
    family, 174
    management, 213–216

tacrine hydrochloride, 61, 66
tai chi, 228
telling people about concerns, 27, 28
temporal lobe, 57
    behaviours affected, 55–56
therapies, alternative, 68–70
therapy *see* counselling/therapy
time and place disorientation, 13–14
treatment options, 47–50
    alternative therapies, 68–70
    doctor and specialist management
      plan, 47–48

drug treatments, 59–70
multidisciplinary approach, 48
rejection of specialist help, 49
specialised care centres, 48–49

Ungunmerr, Miriam-Rose, 237
vascular dementia, 2, 238
vitamins, 69

walking, 229
websites, 258–260
Whittaker, Carl, 148
Wilkinson, Dr Heather, 44
wills, 107, 117
Wilson's disease, 16

Yale, Robin, 90
younger onset dementia, 20–22

Acknowledgments

I would like to acknowledge my profound debt to all the special people who have contributed to this book over the past seven years, both directly as interviewees and indirectly as clients. They are people who have had the courage to seek support, information and counselling for themselves or with a member of the family. I have been privileged to witness the many positive changes that have occurred in their lives and the difference that has made to the way they have lived alongside or with a dementing illness.

Very special thanks go to Jacki King, Noreen Whittaker, Adrienne Sallay, Mary Roddy, Fay Crampton, Narelle Scotford, Barbara Cail and Wendy Cavernett. Each has offered something unique and different that I now understand contributes to the tapestry of writing and the wisdom of life.

Thanks also go to the staff of the Alzheimer's Association in NSW and the ACT. Michelle McGrath deserves a special award for her contributions. Not only did she offer her delightful Canberra home as a venue for interviews, but she also arranged for people with early stage dementia to share their experiences, in the hope that it will help others.

My deep appreciation goes to the essential and dedicated work of my publisher Pam Brewster, Sales and Marketing Director Mary Drum and all the exceptional behind-the-scenes staff at Hodder Headline Australia who have made the publication of this book possible.

Finally, love to my husband Norm who has provided the encouragement and the belief that this endeavour was achievable. And to my daughter Fiona Curtin who thought nothing of driving 800 kilometres for a weekend just to 'be there' for me throughout the writing process.